— SECOND EDITION —

An Encyclopedia
OF NATURAL
HEALING
FOR Children
AND Infants

Mary Bove, N.D.

D1227521

Keats Publishing

Chicago   New York   San Francisco   Lisbon   London   Madrid   Mexico City
Milan   New Delhi   San Juan   Seoul   Singapore   Sydney   Toronto

Library of Congress Cataloging-in-Publication Data

Bove, Mary.
    An encyclopedia of natural healing for children and infants / Mary Bove.—2nd
ed.
        p.   cm.
    Includes bibliographical references and index.
    ISBN 0-658-00725-4
      1. Pediatrics—Popular works.   2. Children—Diseases—Alternative
treatment—Popular works.   3. Naturopathy—Popular works.   I. Title.

RJ61.B7883   2001
618.92—dc21   2001029294

Keats Publishing

A Division of The **McGraw·Hill** Companies

1 2 3 4 5 6 7 8 9 0 DOH/DOH 0 9 8 7 6 5 4 3 2 1

ISBN 0-658-00725-4

This book was set in Sabon
Printed and bound by R. R. Donnelley—Harrisonburg

Cover design by Laurie Young and Barbara Briggs Garibay

McGraw-Hill books are available at special quantity discounts to use as premiums and
sales promotions, or for use in corporate training programs. For more information, please
write to the Director of Special Sales, Professional Publishing, McGraw-Hill, Two Penn
Plaza, New York, NY 10121-2298. Or contact your local bookstore.

An Encyclopedia of Natural Healing for Children and Infants, Second Edition is not intended
as medical advice. Its intention is solely informational and educational. Please consult a
medical or health professional should the need for one be indicated. The information in this
book lends itself to self-help. For obvious reasons, the author and publisher cannot take the
medical or legal responsibility of having the contents herein considered as a prescription for
everyone. Either you or the physician who examines and treats you must take the
responsibility for the uses made of this book.

This book is printed on acid-free paper.

To my children, Amelia and Will—my greatest teachers

Contents

Part V
The Child's Herbal Medicine Chest 201

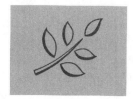

Acknowledgments

I would like to thank the many people who have encouraged and inspired me on my journey in natural medicine, especially my mother, Dorothy M. Bove, who so many years ago introduced me to the magic scent of herbs and planted a seed.

I would like to thank my teachers Norma Myers, Hein Zeylstra, Dr. Louis Bove, and Dr. Molly Linton for their guidance and wisdom in healing. I also want to acknowledge the many children who have brought me healing lessons, particularly all the babies whose births I have been blessed to attend.

Thanks to my children, Amelia and William, for their patience and understanding during my long hours at the computer. Thanks to David for his love, support, humor, and ear during my more anxious moments.

HERBAL BLESSING

In a mountain field
in summer
I am alone among
my herbs.
These plants are my children.

It is hot
so hot, that the air
looks liquid
above seeding plants
that add a gentle percussion
with their bursting
to the music of the humming bees.

Hot summer makes all things golden.

I harvest my herb gifts,
and sing thanks in my heart
for their yielding.

—Mary Bove

Introduction
The Herbal Approach
to Healing

HERBS AND HEALTH CARE

Parents today want to take a more active role in their children's health care; they are looking for safe, effective ways to enhance their children's well-being. They want to be able to treat the occasional cold or tummyache at home or perhaps find an alternative medicine for a health condition that has not responded to traditional allopathic treatment.

Herbal medicine offers a natural approach to health that has been used for hundreds of years by many peoples living all over the earth. Knowledge about the medicinal qualities of plants continues to grow through modern scientific research, which serves to discover new information as well as to confirm empirical information that has been handed down through many different cultures in the traditional medicine systems of the world.

The medical benefits of herbs are vast. They offer safe, natural alternatives that work to rebuild and heal the body. Medicinal herbs can be used to stimulate, support, or calm a body system or area. They can be used as a primary treatment or to complement another type of treatment. They can be used in simple first-aid care, as with an herbal salve to treat a bug bite or scratch, an acute cold or flu, or a chronic condition of the skin or respiratory system. Herbs can aid in the recovery from illness, support the body's immune system, and reduce the side effects of more powerful drugs.

A variety of herbal preparations can be used safely by informed parents in the health care of their infants and children. Often, they are available in health food stores or may be purchased from an herbalist or naturopathic physician. Better yet, many of these preparations can be easily made up in the home and used for conditions such as coughs, colds, flus, or skin rashes, which are usually treated with standard over-the-counter pharmaceuticals. In fact, most natural herbal preparations work as well or even better than the usual drugstore remedies.

Parents can use herbal medicines either preventively—to strengthen immunity or support body functions—or as treatment for a specific illness. Herbs can act as anti-inflammatories, antifungals, antibacterials, or as tissue repairers. They can be applied in a variety of forms, from mild (baths, creams, teas) to strong (tinctures or capsules).

Herbs can be the only medicine used, or they can be used to support other more conventional medications and treatments. For example, an acute strep throat is often treated with an antibiotic medicine that will effectively eradicate the infective agent causing the disease but will not heal the local tissue damage, address the weakness of the immune system, or replace the beneficial digestive flora that the antibiotic destroys. An excellent complementary treatment to be used along with the prescribed antibiotic to augment healing might include yarrow or meadowsweet to reduce inflammation, calendula to increase local tissue repair, and acidophilus supplementation to replace the digestive flora.

Many times, parents first come to my office after their child has suffered from a constantly recurring illness. Such a child typically suffers from repeated ear or upper respiratory infections, skin rashes, or sore throats that do not resolve with the treatments prescribed by the medical doctor and require repeated doses of antibiotics or other pharmaceutical medications.

It is here that alternative health approaches can be most effective. When we look at the body as a whole, with all systems interconnected, each affecting the other, the goal is not merely to treat the symptom but to treat the underlying cause of the symptom. By using herbal medicines to address not only the infective agent but also the immune response in the affected area as well as in the whole body, the cycle of disease can be interrupted. This will then allow the body to grow strong, come into balance, and heal itself.

THE BENEFITS AND SAFETY OF HERBAL MEDICINE FOR INFANTS AND CHILDREN

Infants and children generally respond to herbal medicines easily and positively. Their bodies are smaller and their systems are still maturing, which makes them more vulnerable to the healing effects of mild herbs (as well as to the unwelcome side effects of harsh drugs). Herbal medicines offer safe, effective alternatives that can support and strengthen the body while treating the illness. Most of them can be safely used over a long period of time without any danger of adverse reactions.

When working with infants and children, the form in which the medicine is administered is of great importance. There are many types of herbal preparations to choose from, and often several types of herbal preparations are used to treat one illness.

Many of the gentle topical preparations such as baths, rubs, poultices, creams, and washes can be used effectively with infants and young children who might not comply with oral dosing of medicine. Teas, syrups, glycerites, and herbal popsicles are milder-tasting oral medications than the alcoholic extracts often used by adults or older children. Having the choice of several ways to administer herbs can allow parents to choose a treatment that fits their child's needs and preferences.

Of course, not every child will tolerate all types of medicinal plants, and some common reactions may occur in hypersensitive children. For example, the herb St. John's wort can cause a skin rash with exposure to the sun. Topical medicines can be patch-tested for twenty-four hours if skin sensitivity is a risk. If your child is hypersensitive or allergic, it is wise to be cautious and start with one or two herbs in reduced doses to assess tolerance.

Safety is always a concern when giving any type of medicine, natural or not. Any herb given for the treatment of infants and children is safe when used wisely and with some knowledge of the herb's activity. It is important to know the individual herb and its potential actions and indications. This will ensure safe and effective use. When in doubt, consult a naturopathic physician or professional herbalist.

Many effective herbal home remedies can be used easily and safely. For example, the use of a potato poultice for a bee sting, a carrot neck poultice or a sage gargle for a sore throat, or a cough syrup made from onions may be all that is necessary for a minor ailment or complaint. Home remedies can improve a sick child's comfort level, treat minor ailments that don't require a doctor's attention, and support the healing of the whole body.

Eating fresh, healthy, live foods such as leafy green vegetables, nettle soup, carrots, onions, garlic, and parsley keep the body's immune system strong and healthy. These nutritious foods, which can easily be included in the family diet, support health in an important way.

In herbal tradition, it was not unusual to have fresh herbs prescribed in a soup. These were called *potherbs*. Some traditional potherbs include nettles, wild garlic, dandelion greens, sorrel, and lovage. These nutrient-rich plants, taken as foods, can strengthen the digestive function, support kidney function, and tonify the body. Immune-boosting soups containing herbs such as onions, garlic, ginger, shiitake mushrooms, and mung bean sprouts can be a healthy support during a flu, cold, or gastritis. The frequent use of herbal punches made with fruit juice and herbs, such as nettles, red clover, linden flowers, astragalus, and ginger, can be helpful in keeping little ones healthy during cold season.

Become acquainted with the healing and nourishing world of herbs. It's a wonderful way to nurture your child and keep him or her in a state of radiant health.

Using Herbal Remedies for Infants and Children

CARING FOR YOUR CHILD

As a parent, you know better than anyone when your child is not feeling well. Sometimes there are signs of illness like diarrhea or a fever. Other times there is only a change in the child's behavior to alert you that something is not right. Parents often ask how they can be better prepared to make decisions about their child's health. First, educate yourself by knowing the symptoms and what to do about them. Second, trust your own feelings about the situation, and last, share your concerns with your health care provider. Respiratory diseases account for more than half of all childhood illness. Often, they are easy to diagnose, and most resolve on their own or with natural and herbal medicines.

Children are remarkably tough and have a strong ability to heal themselves and recover from illness. Good nutrition, a health-supportive lifestyle, exercise, and love help their young bodies to preserve this ability.

HERBAL PREPARATIONS AND DOSAGES FOR INFANTS AND CHILDREN

Herbs may be used in numerous forms and preparations when applied as medicines. Many subtle, less well-known preparations may be employed safely and effectively with children, especially with infants and young children, when administration by mouth is problematic. Herbal medicines can be used therapeutically as infusions, syrups, glycerites, steams, powders, baths, body rubs, tinctures, tablets, and capsules. Often, a warm bath with calming herbs or a warm rub of essential oils applied to the chest to relieve the spasm of a cough is just the right medicine for an uncomfortable, congested child who can't fall asleep. The combination of several herbal preparations can also be effective in treating an illness.

Baths

An herbal bath is an effective way to deliver medicines to an infant or young child. The child must soak in the bath of herbs for a minimum of 15 minutes to hydrate the skin before he or she can begin to absorb the medicinal qualities of the bath. The bath also offers the hydrotherapeutic value of warm water on the body's nervous and immune systems. Baths can be used in the treatment of colds, dehydration, fever, flu, sleeplessness, and muscle injury. Bathing the hands or feet is a great way to treat a young person who does not want to drink medicine. The hands or feet are soaked in an infusion or decoction for 5 to 10 minutes, twice a day. The skin absorbs the herbal medicine, and by nerve reflex it affects the rest of the body.

Body Rubs

A body rub can be an effective way to decrease muscle spasm in the chest (such as with a spastic bronchial cough), back (for skeletal muscle pain), and stomach (for colic or constipation). A rub can also be used to stimulate nerve tissue in the peripheral nervous system and to prevent fluid loss from the skin. Aromatic herbs such as basil, lavender, rosemary, thyme, and wintergreen are often used. Some body rubs may combine an herbal oil with a tincture.

Capsules and Tablets

Capsules and tablets can be convenient methods of administration if the child is able to swallow them. Due to the compliance factor, these kinds of herbal preparations are most commonly used with older children, ages eight to twelve. They allow the ingestion of unpleasant-tasting herbs that may otherwise have to be avoided because of their taste. There are many types of herbal capsules and tablets on the market.

Creams and Ointments

Creams and ointments are easy-to-use topical preparations that offer a wide variety of therapeutic uses for ailments such as skin rashes, burns, cuts and wounds, stings, boils, and sprains.

Fomentations and Poultices

Fomentations and poultices are topical preparations mainly used to treat skin rashes and conditions such as swelling of the muscles, ligaments, or glands, such as tonsils.

Glycerines

Glycerine extracts are becoming very popular herbal medicines for children because of their high plant-sugar content. Most children find them easier to tolerate than alcoholic extracts. They can be used as straight glycerites or can be mixed with tinctures, juices, or teas.

Infusions

Infusions or herbal teas can be pleasant ways to treat as well as to administer fluids to the sick child. Teas can be taken alone or mixed with honey, fruit juice, or frozen into an herbal popsicle for sore throats and gums. Teas for infants can be diluted and given by teaspoon doses, eyedropper, or bottle.

Powders

Herbal powders are used topically to keep the skin dry and free of excess moisture. They can be used to promote skin healing as well as for their antiseptic qualities. They relieve skin rash, diaper rash, and fungal infections of the skin.

Steams

Herbal steams are used to deliver the medicinal qualities of herbs to the upper respiratory system. They tend to warm and decongest the mucous membranes of the nose, sinuses, and throat. Aromatic herbs are most commonly used for the medicinal qualities of the volatile oils contained in them.

Suppositories and Enemas

Suppositories and enemas have the advantage of being absorbed directly into the bloodstream, skipping the oral route and thereby avoiding the unpleasant taste of the herbs being administered.

Syrups

Syrups are pleasant ways to prescribe herbal medicines for children, as they are sweet and easy to take. Syrups may be used with infusions and decoctions of medicinal herbs, or they can be mixed with an unpleasant-tasting herbal tincture to mask the flavor.

Tinctures

Tinctures or alcoholic extracts are more difficult to administer to children because of their taste. Often, they are a necessary part of an herbal formula, as the alcohol base extracts the medicinal plant constituent efficiently. Mixing a tincture with a base of syrup or glycerite is a good way to dilute the tincture and make a better-tasting preparation.

Dosages

When referring to a recommended adult dose, it is necessary to adjust the dosage to a suitable amount for an infant or child. This allows for consideration of age, size, weight, and safety. Generally, with an infant, herbal teas are given in teaspoon doses, 3 to 5 times a day; herbal extracts are given in doses of 5 to 10 drops,

3 times a day; and herbal teas are diluted 1 part water to 1 part tea. Dosages for children can be figured according to age, as shown by the formulas below:

Young's Formula

$$\frac{\text{Age in years}}{\text{Age} + 12} = \text{portion of adult dose}$$

For example, the correct dose for a six-year-old child would be:

$$\frac{6}{6 + 12} = \frac{6}{18} = \frac{1}{3} \text{ of adult dose}$$

Dilling's Formula

$$\frac{\text{Age in years}}{20} = \text{portion of adult dose}$$

Again, for a six-year-old child:

$$\frac{6}{20} = \frac{3}{10} \text{ of adult dose}$$

Duration

How often to give the medicine is also a key to successful treatment. I recommend giving herbal remedies for long-term or chronic conditions 3 times a day, usually with meals. If the condition is acute—such as a fever, sore throat, or flu—I recommend taking the dose more frequently, such as 5 times a day or every 2 hours. This allows for a more rigorous use of the herb to support the body's immune response. It is always wise to continue use of the herbal medicine at a 3-times-a-day dose for 5 to 7 days post-acute phase. This helps to prevent relapse or further complications. Often, a child feels better before the body has totally resolved the illness.

ADMINISTERING HERBAL MEDICINES

Giving herbal medicines to children can be a difficult job at times. Usually this applies to oral administration of herbal preparations, yet even putting a drop into the ear or a cream onto the skin can sometimes be difficult. Let the child know that you are giving medicines. Establish a routine or ritual around the process. Letting the child participate in the process can be constructive. Also, communicate with your child the importance of taking the medicines. Treatment failures are often due to the inadequate administration of the herbal medicines.

When choosing an herbal medicine, it is important to consider your child and his or her personal habits, not just the condition or illness. Try to choose a form of preparation that will fit into your life as well as be acceptable to your child. Often, several types can be used, such as a topical preparation along with internal administration of a medicine. For children, an important consideration is how the medicine tastes. If the mixture of herbs is not pleasant, it is unlikely that the child will take the medicine. Herbs that may help improve a preparation's taste are always a good addition. These include anise, lemon balm, peppermint, stevia, and fennel. Using syrups made from fresh herbs, onions, and garlic in a raw sugar or honey base to flavor the remedy can also improve the taste. Onion or garlic syrup is excellent for coughs and respiratory infections, whether used alone or added to a mixture of tinctures or infusions. Extractions made with a glycerine base are also tasty. Many of the herbs listed in Part V impart their active constituents to glycerine and can be effective in tincture mixtures because of their flavor and their medicinal action. If the child can swallow capsules or tablets, then taste is not a factor.

You can help your child learn to swallow a capsule by coating it with olive oil, yogurt, or maple syrup. Place it on the back of the tongue and give with water, juice, or herbal tea.

A NATURAL FIRST-AID KIT

Herbs and other natural remedies can be used as first aid to relieve minor injuries like cuts, scrapes, bee stings, bug bites, motion sickness, burns, food poisoning, infections, and the first signs of illness, as with fever. Having a first-aid kit ready to go will put you one step ahead when a situation arises. Include remedies to meet all types of first-aid situations along with such items as sterile gauze pads and rolls, adhesive bandages like Band-Aids, adhesive tape, small scissors, Ace bandage wrap, thermometer, tweezers, matches, cotton balls, cotton swabs, and a penlight. Get a sewing box, tackle box, or small plastic case to keep your kit organized and be sure that all the items are labeled with the name of the remedy and its main use. This way, other people will be able to work with your first-aid kit if you are not on hand. My children are familiar with most of the uses of the remedies we carry. Here are some of the remedies I carry in my family's first-aid travel kit.

Rescue Remedy

This is a combination of five Bach Flower remedies that in combination are useful for their effects in trauma, injuries, shock, burns, accidents, and emotional upsets. It may be applied topically in a cream form to painful, swollen, burned, or wounded areas of the body. The remedies include star of Bethlehem, rock rose, impatiens, cherry plum, and clematis. I use it in first-aid situations, ranging from burns, stings, cuts, bumps, falls, broken bones, bad news, first day of school jitters, presurgery, and fever. Give 4 to 5 drops as needed.

Homeopathic Remedies

Apis 6c: Keep this on hand for bee stings, bug bites, and allergic reactions of the skin and respiratory system. Give 4 pellets under the tongue and repeat in 15 minutes. Then use 2 to 3 doses for a day or 2 if the bite is severe.

Arnica 6c: Use for all shocks and injuries; it should be the first remedy given. Use for pain, bleeding, or swelling caused by the injury. Give 3 to 4 pellets, 3 to 5 times a day.

Belladonna 6c: Keep this on hand for fevers that come on suddenly, with reddening of the face and lots of heat radiating from the skin. Give 4 pellets and repeat in 15 to 30 minutes.

Cantharis 6c: Use this immediately after a burn to lessen the severity and to help in the healing. Give 3 to 4 pellets every few hours after the burn and 3 times a day for a few days following.

Chamomilla 6c: Keep this on hand for the teething blues, fever, irritability, one cheek reddened, or for a child who needs lots of comfort. Give 2 pellets every 30 minutes in acute episodes or 3 times a day with milder symptoms.

Rhus tox 6c: Keep this on hand for treating poison ivy, poison oak, or poison sumac. Give 4 pellets at the first sign of exposure or rash. Repeat several times a day until rash is resolved.

Herbal First-Aid Remedies

Composition Essence for Children (available from Gaia's Children): Composition Essence has a long history in herbal medicine, being first compounded by Samuel Thomson, the father of Thomsonian medicine. The compound acts as a powerful stimulant, astringent, and tonic. Thomson recommends this composition for the first stages of illness. Traditionally, this formula was given as a hot drink, using the hot water to aid in raising the body's temperature and stimulating circulation, sweating, and an immune response. A pleasant-tasting hot drink can be made by adding ½ cup of boiling water to ½ cup of apple, grape, or berry juice and the appropriate dose of Composition Essence for Children (see label). Drink warm 3 to 4 times a day and keep the child warm. Use for complaints of fever, flu, colds, coughs, earaches, nasal congestions, sore throats, chills, stomachaches, asthma attacks, constipation, and muscle ache.

Fever Drops: This is a mixture of linden flowers, meadowsweet, chamomile flowers, elder flowers, and spearmint leaves in a base of elder and ginger syrup. It is particularly effective when given at the first sign of fever. Give ¼ to ½ teaspoon in ½ cup of hot water and bundle the child up. (A good product is Elder/Ginger drops by Gaia Herbs.)

Yarrow-Calendula Antiseptic Drops: To prepare, mix ½ ounce each of the tinctures of yarrow flowers and calendula flowers.

Add 30 drops of this mixture to 1 tablespoon of water and use to wash cuts, stings, bites, or scrapes.

Ginger Drops for nausea, motion sickness, or indigestion: Add ½ teaspoon of ginger tincture to a 1-ounce dropper bottle and fill with filtered water. Use 5 to 10 drops on the tongue, as needed for discomfort.

Echinacea Ginger Drops: Add ½ teaspoon of ginger tincture to a 1-ounce dropper bottle and fill the rest with echinacea glycerite. Use ½ teaspoon in a cup of warm water as a gargle for sore throats or as a tea for flu, colds, fever, and infections. Give 3 to 4 times a day.

Creams and Salves

Arnica Cream can be used for all types of bruising, swelling, sprains, and strains. This can be applied topically to the area several times a day.

Calendula Comfrey Salve makes an excellent all-purpose salve for all types of cuts, scrapes, burns, bites, stings, rashes, sunburn, and chapped lips.

Other First-Aid Remedies

Acetaminophen (e.g., Tylenol) or **ibuprofen** (e.g., Advil)

Benadryl: an over-the-counter antihistamine

Insect repellent: See Insect Bites, page 148.

Vitamin C, chewable or powder: Give a dose after all types of physical trauma. Use for fevers, infections, and flu. Also can be given for constipation to increase bowel tolerance while traveling.

Vitamin E: This can be used orally for burns and bleeding. Use 400 I.U. to 800 I.U., as needed. It can also be used topically for all types of skin rash, bites, burns, cuts, and sprains.

PART

II

Working with the Young Immune System

Every parent wants a healthy child. Good health depends on a healthy immune system. A healthy, efficient immune system is the key to a healthy, happy child who will resist infection, allergy, and chronic illness. The job of the immune system is to protect and defend the body against infection from disease-producing micro-organisms such as the viruses, bacteria, fungi, and parasites that live in our environment. When the immune system is healthy and functioning properly, it fights off the micro-organisms and sets up a healing response to repair the damage. Often, the body never shows any sign of the fight. At other times the signs of illness are present.

BASIC IMMUNE SYSTEM MECHANICS

The immune system has several mechanisms for defending and protecting the body. Some of the basic barrier mechanisms include secretions of the eye, nose, mouth, stomach, skin, and mucous membranes. The major components of the immune system are the lymphatic vessels and organs, including the tonsils, adenoids, lymph nodes, thymus gland, spleen, white blood cells, and specialized cells residing in various tissues, such as macrophages and mast cells.

When an infectious agent enters the body, an inflammatory response is set up, which causes the small blood vessels to dilate and increase the flow of blood and thus bring more white blood cells to the damaged area. Cells around the damaged area secrete substances, including histamine, to cause the white blood cells to move from the bloodstream to the damaged site. If still more defense is necessary, other white blood cells appear, called monocytes, which attack the micro-organisms even more aggressively. Next, the lymphatic system will start to move debris and micro-organisms to the lymph nodes, where more concentrated amounts of white blood cells reside. Here, macrophages eat up the micro-organisms and debris, and the lymphocytes begin to produce antibodies to the invading micro-organisms. When the body is under attack, the lymph nodes often enlarge as more lymphocytes are produced to defend the body, such as when a child gets swollen glands with a sore throat.

The two main types of lymphocytes are B-cells and T-cells. T-cells mature in the thymus gland and consist of several types. Killer T-cells attack infected cells with a cell poison, helper T-cells communicate with the B-cells to call them into action, and T-suppressor cells control the action of the other lymphocytes and stop the mechanism when the infection has been resolved.

B-cells mature in the bone marrow and produce antibodies to bind to specific antigens. Once this has occurred, a B-memory cell is produced that will stimulate immunity in the future against the same particular micro-organisms.

The lymphatic organs play a major role in immune-system functioning. In children and infants, the thymus gland plays an important part in the development of immunity. The gland is located at the base of the throat and is much larger in children than in adults, as it shrinks in size with age. The thymus gland's primary function is to produce T-lymphocytes, whose job includes producing antibodies against viruses and infected cells. Other lymphatic organs include the spleen, liver, tonsils, and adenoids. The digestive tract is also lined with lymphatic tissue. This is one of the major routes of contact with foreign substances, so good digestive immune functioning is essential to good health. It follows then that healthy digestive functioning is also essential to good health.

It is important to remember that an infant's immune system is immature at birth. Fortunately, however, a newborn carries passive immunity from the mother for the first three months of life. It has been shown that breast-feeding helps to provide the infant with maternal antibodies and immune-enhancing factors to help build immunity. A baby's lymphocytes are not yet capable of producing all the antibodies necessary to fight disease. A baby acquires this ability during the first year of life. As the infant is exposed to micro-organisms, the lymphocytes start to make antibodies and memory cells so that when the baby comes into contact with those micro-organisms again the body will mount an immune response more quickly.

BUILDING A HEALTHY IMMUNE SYSTEM

Healthy development of the immune system depends on good nutrition to provide the body with the essential building blocks needed for the defense system.

Proteins are essential as a source of the amino acids needed as building blocks for the immune tissue and organs and for antibody production.

Essential fatty acids (EFAs) are especially important to a healthy immune system. They are crucial to the normal functioning of lymphocytes and the production of antibodies. They are used to build a healthy, functional cell membrane around every cell in the body; they are needed as building blocks for endocrine hormones as well as tissue prostaglandins; and they are necessary for the healthy functioning of the heart, kidneys, blood, and nervous system, including brain function.

Vitamin A is vital in the production of T- and B-cells, which are the main antibody-producing white blood cells. Vitamin A is needed for healthy lymph tissue and lymphatic function and for building a strong thymus and spleen.

Beta-carotene, which is found in orange, yellow, and green vegetables, is a powerful antioxidant and is important in immune function and mucous membrane health.

Vitamin B6 is necessary for healthy mucous membranes, a key line of defense against the external environment. B6 is also used by the immune system to produce B- and T-lymphocytes. B6 requires the presence of zinc, a cofactor that helps the vitamin to be utilized by the body and have a full effect on mucous membrane health.

Vitamin C acts as a nutrient as well as a strong antioxidant in the body, quieting the breakdown of body tissue. It plays a big part in defending the body from bacteria and viruses, stimulates macrophage activity to eat up invading micro-organisms, and encourages antibody response and killer T-cell production.

Vitamin E is a powerful antioxidant that reduces cell damage by reducing free radical activity and maintaining homeostasis in the white blood cells. It enhances the production of antibodies and macrophages and aids in enhancing the immune system's resistance to viruses. The mineral selenium seems to enhance the effects of vitamin E.

Magnesium is a key mineral in the metabolism of EFAs into prostaglandins, hormone-like substances that help to regulate the activity of the white blood cells. Diets that are high in preserved refined foods and artificial substances tend to be deficient in magnesium.

Zinc is probably the most vital mineral to a healthy immune system. It is involved in T-cell production, in tissue healing and repair, and has a strong antiviral activity. It plays an important role in the utilization of B6 in immune health. Zinc gets into our food from the soil. Thus, poor-quality soil and artificial fertilizers lower the zinc level in many fruits and vegetables. Diets that are high in milk and cheese are often low in zinc.

Selenium is a micromineral that acts as an antioxidant in the body, reducing free radical activity and eliminating heavy metals, such as lead and mercury, from the body. Selenium enhances the activity of macrophages, increases the production of antibodies, and increases the T-cell's ability to destroy bacteria.

Bioflavonoid compounds are found in green plants and many fruits. They enhance the effects of vitamin C as a therapeutic agent, have antiviral activity, stabilize mast cells, and prevent free radical damage to muscles, joints, blood vessels, and many other organs.

Coenzyme Q10 has recently been recognized as an immune-building agent, important in fighting infection. It enhances the energy produced in the immune cells, increasing immune activity. CoQ10 provides antioxidant activity against free radical damage. This nutrient is found in broccoli, spinach, sardines, mackerel, and eggs.

All of these essential nutrients can be found in a diet rich in organic fresh fruits and vegetables, good whole-grain fibers, and good-quality fats and oils. A diet low in saturated fats, refined processed foods, refined sugars, and additives will help to support good immune system development by providing the needed nutrients.

FOODS THAT WEAKEN THE IMMUNE SYSTEM

The following foods tend to have little nutritional value, and they weaken the immune system by blocking the essential fatty acids' function in the body. These foods are antinutrients and actually antagonize nutrients needed for health by binding to them and rendering them useless. These antinutrients also use up the enzymes needed for digestion and other body systems, they increase the need for certain nutrients, and they cause some nutrients to be excreted from the body. EFAs play an important role in good immune function and general health, and it is essential to provide an adequate supply in the diet as well as to avoid substances that interrupt their metabolism and function in the body. This is why it is not only important to minimize antinutrient foods in a child's diet but also to provide the body with a variety of vitamins and minerals that will help it deal with poor-quality foods.

Sugars: A diet high in refined sugars will weaken the work of EFAs in the body. Sugar increases the loss of magnesium and other minerals in the urine and depletes the body of B vitamins, leading to a weakened immune response.

Nonessential Fatty Acids/Poor Fats: These types of fats, including hydrogenated oils, margarine, and fried fats, block EFA metabolism and compete for the enzymes used by EFAs. This leads to immune dysfunction and free radical damage. Unhealthy fats will destroy cell membranes. They will also produce substances in the body that create more tissue breakdown and unfavorable prostaglandins.

Processed Preserved Foods and Soda: Foods that are processed contain large amounts of sodium and phosphates. Sodium found naturally in whole foods is adequate to fill the body's needs. The amount of sodium found in processed preserved foods is much more than the body needs. Increased levels of sodium cause magnesium, potassium, and other crucial cofactors to be lost in the urine. High levels of phosphates in the body disrupt good bowel absorption of nutrients such as calcium and magnesium. This can lead to problems in EFA metabolism, muscle and bone development, and cardiovascular health. Soft drinks and soda pop are very high in phosphates and are best avoided altogether.

Pesticides: Modern agriculture uses many pesticides and herbicides in the mass growing of fruits, vegetables, and grains. Their residues remain on most foods to some degree and interfere with the use of vitamin B6 as a cofactor in the body. B6 deficiency can lead to poor EFA metabolism, dysfunction in blood sugar regulation, and a range of neurological conditions. Choose organic produce whenever possible.

FREE RADICAL THEORY

Free radicals are highly reactive molecules found in the body that bind and destroy cell membranes and other cellular components. Free radicals come from external sources such as X rays, sunlight, chemicals, tobacco, and certain foods. Internally, they occur dur-

 Free Radical Sources Found in the Environment

- Sunlight
- X rays
- Radiation
- Pesticides
- Air pollutants
- Petroleum-based products such as Vaseline
- Solvents like formaldehyde
- Furniture polish
- Cleaning products
- Paints
- Alcohol
- Tobacco
- Fried, barbecued, and smoked foods
- Margarine and hydrogenated vegetable oils
- Coffee
- Heavy metals such as lead and mercury

ing chemical reactions. Exposure to external and dietary free radicals will increase the free radical load in the body and lead to tissue breakdown. Reducing one's exposure to these substances adds to a healthier immune system and a happier child.

IMMUNE SYSTEM MALFUNCTION

When the immune system fights the battle against infection, it either wins or loses. If it is the first exposure to the micro-organism, as with measles, mumps, or chicken pox, or if the immune system is compromised, the micro-organism will win. Modern medicine uses antibiotics and vaccinations to help the body mount an immune response. This has reduced the incidence of acute childhood diseases such as polio, measles, diphtheria, and whooping cough. However, we are only now beginning to see the long-term effects of this medical approach.

The overprescription of antibiotics is a big contributing factor to many chronic health problems. Overprescribing often occurs between the ages of one and six years old, when there is a high incidence of ear infection. Many times, antibiotic treatment is not necessary but is prescribed anyway. The long-term results of repeated antibiotic use can lead to urinary tract infections and compromise of the intestinal microflora. This sets up a risk of malabsorption and food allergy. When treating a child for chronic bladder infections, I always need to address associated yeast overgrowth or food allergy because of the likelihood of prior repeated antibiotic use.

Antibiotics and the Immune System

Antibiotics resolve infectious diseases, save lives, reduce suffering, and will continue to do so. Yet the overprescribing and the misuse of these medicines have led to problems of their own. The health problems associated with antibiotic use, such as a rise in secondary infections after antibiotic treatment, are just beginning to become apparent. Some of these include:

- **Antibiotic-resistant bacteria.** These bacteria develop in response to repeated antibiotic use and lead to stronger, more virulent strains of the bacteria, which a child may harbor and which may persist with chronic symptoms of illness. Antibiotic treatment has also led nondisease-causing bacteria to mutate into more virulent strains and become disease causing, as with the bacteria *E. coli*.
- **Destruction of friendly bacteria.** There are hundreds of friendly bacteria living in the body, helping to protect against unfriendly bacteria. *Lactobacillus* bacteria are among the many friendly bacteria living in the intestinal tract. These bacteria are diminished by the use of antibiotics, which do not differentiate between friendly and nonfriendly bacteria. That is why it is always a good idea to use an acidophilus supplement when taking antibiotics.
- **Antibiotics and yeast.** Antibiotic treatment has been associated with yeast overgrowth, such as thrush developing in a baby after antibiotic treatment. Overgrowth of yeast in the body leads to suppression of the immune system and a greater risk of developing illness.
- **Antibiotics and immune suppression.** While antibiotics are intended to bolster the immune response by killing bacteria, they may also have a suppressive effect on the immune system, particularly with repeated use. Treatment with antibiotics can often increase the likelihood of a repeat infection. My goal is to avoid the use of antibiotics as much as possible but, if they must be used, to accompany them with good immune support through vitamins, minerals, and herbs.

- **Nutrient loss.** Antibiotics can contribute to the loss of vital nutrients needed by the immune system to fight infection. The loss may occur because of digestive irritation, diarrhea, or dysfunctional intestinal flora.
- **Allergic reaction to antibiotics.** Various allergic reactions are often associated with antibiotic therapy. Common side effects of antibiotics include skin rash, hives, diarrhea, and swelling of the throat. These symptoms may be due to the drug itself or the wide variety of chemicals and dyes used in the manufacturing of the medicines.

Allergic Reaction and the Immune System

The immature immune system develops the ability to not only fight foreign micro-organisms but also recognize the body and all that belongs to it. Sometimes, the immune system gets confused and attacks the body's own tissues and organs, creating what is called an autoimmune response. When the immune system attacks harmless or even beneficial substances, such as foods or pollens, it is called an allergic response. An allergic reaction is an exaggerated immune response to a substance. Allergy-stimulating substances can be natural or artificial, including foods, pollens, mildew, mold, chemicals, smoke, and so on. The signs and symptoms produced by the allergic response are caused by the release of chemicals such as histamine. Mast cells, which are found in the mucous membranes of the respiratory system, digestive system, and all other mucous membranes, produce antibodies called immunoglobulins. Immunoglobulins bind to the mast cells and form a complex with the allergen. Because they have a memory, they will act this way every time that particular allergen is present. When these complexes are formed, chemicals such as histamine and inflammatory prostaglandins are released, causing such symptoms as swelling of the mucous membranes,

Common Symptoms of Allergic Reaction

- Asthma
- Eczema
- Hay fever
- Headaches
- Hives
- Dry or rough skin and skin rash
- Chronic runny nose, nasal congestion, or sinusitis
- Frequent respiratory infections, coughs, earaches, tonsillitis, and chronic colic
- Chronic diarrhea or constipation
- Food cravings or fussy eating
- Tiredness and fatigue
- Behavioral problems, restlessness, and hyperactivity
- Learning problems and poor concentration
- Poor sleep patterns
- Bed-wetting
- Muscle and joint pain

overproduction of mucus, nasal congestion, irritation of the eyes, asthma, hives, eczema, inflammation of the intestines, and diarrhea. The allergic reaction is the body's effort to get rid of a substance it feels is potentially harmful.

A child will present with different types of allergic symptoms depending on family history, age, and general immune system health. If a child has a parent or sibling with an allergy and the child is also allergic, it is often to the same types of things. An allergic response can vary depending on age. Babies tend to react to things that touch their skin, such as diapers, lotions, soaps, laundry detergents, nylon or wool, or things they are eating such as formula, foods, and substances in the breast milk like dairy products or drugs. Toddlers tend to react to the same things as babies, in addition to the infectious agents they become infected by. Older children react to all of these as well as to airborne allergens such as dust, dander, molds, pollens, and chemicals. Older children develop more respiratory symptoms, similar to an adult.

Food Allergy

Food allergy or food intolerance is very common in the United States and has been on the rise over the last two decades. Some theories as to why there is an increased incidence of food intolerance include an increased stress load on the immune system

Systems and Symptoms Associated with Food Allergies

Digestive: Gas, diarrhea, colic, canker sores, constipation, irritable colon, or irregular stool pattern
Urinary: Bed-wetting or chronic bladder infection
Respiratory: Chronic earache, runny nose, sinusitis, wheezing, chronic bronchitis, or itchy nose, ears, and throat
Immune: Chronic repeated infections
Skin: Acne, eczema, hives, or itchy skin
Muscles: Painful joints, back pain, muscle spasm, or headache
Mental: Migraine headaches, depression, or anxiety
Emotional: Hyperactivity, poor concentration, or insomnia

from pollutants, chemicals, foods, and water; earlier weaning and the premature introduction of solid foods to infants; and less variety in foods eaten. Symptoms of food intolerance may be mild to debilitating and may occur immediately after ingesting the offending food. However, the majority of symptoms are delayed and show up over several days, making food allergy identification more difficult. The reaction can be caused by a food protein, starch, or any food component, or a contaminant such as food coloring or a preservative. Many reactions express themselves in many forms and in many different areas of the body. The following are common signs of food allergy:

- Dark circles under the eyes
- Puffiness under the eyes
- Horizontal creases in the lower eyelid
- Chronic swollen glands
- Chronic postnasal drip
- Chronic noncyclic fluid retention

Causes of Food Allergy

Genetic predisposition. A food allergy is often the expression of an inherited genetic predisposition. Often, food allergies are shared by other family members. The expression of the allergy

 Diseases Associated with Food Allergy

- Asthma
- Colitis
- Celiac disease
- Kidney disease

can be triggered by a variety of stresses, including physical and emotional trauma, excessive drug use, immunization reaction, or an excessive and frequent intake of high-allergen foods. On the other hand, the expression of an immune-mediated food allergy is caused by the interaction among the ingested food antigens, digestive tract, histamine, white blood cells, and immune compounds.

Immune system disorder. An immune system disorder is sometimes the cause of a food allergy. The dysfunction occurs in the T-cell lymphocyte activity, which leads to an increase in allergy reactivity. Nonimmunological mechanisms are triggered by inflammation rather than an antibody. Inflammatory mediators like prostaglandins and histamine can cause allergic response.

Malabsorption, poor digestion, repeated food exposure, and poor integrity of the intestinal wall. All of these disorders affect the development of a food allergy. It has been shown that partially digested dietary protein can cross the intestinal wall and be taken into the body. Factors that can increase intestinal wall permeability include abnormal gut flora, decrease in normal gut flora, immunity of the digestive tract, low levels of pancreatic digestive enzymes, decrease in stomach acid, vitamin A deficiency, chronic diarrhea, and inflammation of the digestive tract.

These foods are likely to cause allergy:

- Milk products
- Wheat
- Eggs
- Citrus fruits and drinks
- Soy
- Corn
- Gluten

- Chocolate, tea, and coffee
- Peanuts and peanut butter
- Food additives and colorings
- Refined sugars
- Tomatoes
- Shellfish

Treatment of Food Allergy

The key to working with allergies is not only to identify the allergen but also to consider all other factors that compromise the proper functioning of the immune system. If the allergen is removed and the immune system continues to malfunction, then there is a very good chance that the child will start to react to some other allergen over time. The whole treatment consists not only of avoiding the allergens but also improving the functioning of the digestive system and immune system and correcting nutritional deficiencies.

Identifying and eliminating the offending food or foods from the diet can eliminate stress on the body and allow the body to heal. Foods to suspect are those that are commonly known allergens (see preceding list) or foods that the child ingests daily or even craves. Try eliminating these foods from the child's diet for one to two weeks. Watch to see if any of the allergic symptoms change during this time. Then add the foods back one at a time, a new one every three days. Watch to see if symptoms worsen or return. If you find a symptom that is linked to a certain food, avoid that food, and use herbal and nutritional medicines to improve digestive and immune system function. In a younger child, the longer a food is eliminated from the diet, the more likely the child will be able to tolerate it in moderate amounts later. Try to keep the child off the offending food for at least three months. When reintroducing a food into the diet, add it only a few times a week and never let the child eat it daily. Rotating foods in the diet so that they are not repeated daily can help to increase the foods a sensitive child can eat. It is not always easy to tell exactly what foods a child will react to. In this case avoid the most common food allergens for several months.

Nutritional supplementation of immune-strengthening vitamins and minerals can reduce histamine, decrease inflammation, boost the immune response, and improve the vitality of the mucous membranes. Use buffered vitamin C, 250 milligrams to 500 milligrams, 4 times a day, for its antihistamine and decongestant effects; bioflavonoids for the antiallergic action (quercitin, 300 milligrams, 2 to 3 times a day); beta-carotene and zinc for the membranes and immune response; and essential fatty acids. (See Part III for doses.)

Disturbances of the digestive tract, such as low growth of microflora, digestive enzyme dysfunctions, constipation, irritation, and inflammation of the stomach or intestines, may all contribute to allergic tendencies. Give acidophilus between meals, 1 to 2 caps or ½ to 1 teaspoon per dose, 2 to 3 times per day. Use digestive plant enzymes with meals to help the system digest the food and lessen the strain on it. Address constipation, chronic diarrhea, or inflammatory disease of the intestines if present. (See Part IV.)

Nettles in the freeze-dried capsulated form can be given, 2 capsules, 3 times a day. They act to reduce the allergic reaction, reduce histamine in the body, and strengthen the body's resistance. Select herbs in tea or extract form to build up the immune system and reduce the allergic immune response. The appropriate herbs are astragalus, chamomile flowers, elder flowers, eyebright, echinacea, licorice, nettles, and red clover.

Nutrition for Infants and Children

Producing healthy children is one of the most important roles we have as parents. A diet high in good-quality foods will provide the nutrients children need to grow and stay healthy. The first year of life is characterized by rapid physical growth and development. The adequacy of the infant's nutritional intake will have an effect on how the infant interacts with his or her environment. Healthy, well-nourished babies have the energy to respond to and learn from the stimuli in their environment and interact and bond with their parents. There is a slower growth pattern in the time from one year of age to puberty than in the first year of life. In general, most preschool and school-age children experience a steady physical growth pattern and a rapid growth in cognitive functioning, language, and social skills. Children at this age are often very particular about the foods they eat. Often, it is difficult to get them to eat a balanced, nutritional diet. Thus, supplementation with a good multiple vitamin and mineral can be a helpful way to ensure an adequate amount of essential nutrients are integrated into your child's diet. Vitamin and mineral supplements are best taken with meals.

HEALTH AND THE ROLE OF THE DIGESTIVE SYSTEM

Proper digestion is a requirement for good health and immunity. Incomplete or dysfunctional digestion can be a major contributor to the development of food allergies and many diseases. Not only are undigested foods and nutrients of little value when breakdown and assimilation are inadequate, but incompletely digested food molecules can be inappropriately absorbed into the body. Regardless of how nutritious the food is, the body must absorb it for it to have any nutritional value. To absorb it, the digestive organs and bowel microflora must also be functioning well.

The digestive tract is made up of the mouth, esophagus, stomach, small intestine (which has three different parts), large intestine, and colon. Supportive organs for the digestive system are the liver and pancreas, which provide important secretions for the breakdown of food. The microflora of the intestines also play an important part in digestive health. These micro-organisms help to regulate digestive pH, protect from the overgrowth of undesirable bacteria, aid in the breakdown of food particles, and play a role in immune defense. Because the digestive system interfaces with our outside environment through the food we eat, our system is lined with immune tissues to help protect the body from toxins. This creates a strong connection between immune health and a healthy digestive system.

When a baby is born, the digestive system is still immature. It lacks the ability to digest certain foods and food groups. Over the first twelve to eighteen months, the baby's digestive tract matures and becomes able to deal with all types of food. If the baby is exposed to food substances and proteins before the digestive system is able to process these molecules, there is a potential for the child's body to trigger an antibody reaction. The antibody can then stay in the circulation, and the next time that food is ingested it will trigger an immune response. Common food allergies can cause symptoms that include colic, constipation, diarrhea, gas, bloating, skin rash, eczema, recurrent respiratory infections, ear infections, asthma, tonsillitis, mood swings, behavioral problems, and irritability. To complicate the matter even further, once the body has become intolerant of a food, continued ingestion of the offending food can trigger intolerance to other foods. This is due to the infant's gut membrane, which becomes more permeable to substances, resulting in the "leaky gut" syndrome. Common foods causing these reactions are cow's milk and products, eggs, corn, wheat, citrus, and peanuts. One can see how important it is for good health that a child's digestive tract be working well. When foods are introduced too early, particularly high-risk allergic foods, or the child has been treated often with antibiotics, the digestion is going to be compromised.

Ensuring good digestive function through good-quality foods, chewing foods well, eating when relaxed, and not overeating will contribute to the body's general health and defense system and decrease the risk of chronic disease.

ESSENTIAL NUTRIENTS

Proteins

Proteins are essential for growth, repair, and maintenance of all body tissues. They act as building blocks for hormones, antibodies, immune compounds, enzymes, and neurotransmitters. Proteins are broken down in the body into amino acids, some of which are used to make other amino acids. Adequate protein intake is essential for proper growth and physiological development in a child. Protein sources are classified as primary or secondary. Primary protein sources are meats, poultry, fish, eggs, milk, and soy products. Secondary sources are nuts, seeds, nut butters, legumes, whole grains, and sprouted grains. Small amounts of protein are also found in fruits and vegetables.

PROTEIN CONTENT OF FOODS

Food	Grams of Protein
Almonds, ¼ cup	7.3
Beans or lentils, ½ cup	3.0
Beef, 3 ounces	22.0
Broccoli, 1 cup, cooked	8.0
Brown rice, ½ cup	4.0
Carrot	1.1
Cheese, hard 1½ ounces	11.0
Chicken, 3 ounces	26.0
Cottage cheese, ⅔ cup	20.5
Dried figs, 2	2.2
Egg, 1	6.5
Milk, 1 cup	8.5
Peanut butter, 1 tablespoon	3.9
Potato, 8 ounces	5.0
Salmon, 3 ounces	17.0
Soy milk, 1 cup	8.0
Tofu, 3 ounces	8.0
Tahini, 1 tablespoon	2.5

Whole-grain bread, 1 slice   1.2
Whole-wheat pasta, ¾ cup   10.0
Yogurt, ½ cup   6.5

PROTEIN RDA FOR CHILDREN

Age	Grams per Day
1–3	25
4–6	30
7–10	35

Vegetarian children can consume an adequate amount of dietary protein if the daily diet includes a wide variety of organic, unrefined foods. The use of fortified rice, soy, or nut milk can provide more protein. The use of protein powders made from milk, soy, or rice can be added to cereals, baked goods, or sauces to increase the protein value of the meal. Supplementation with shakes made with fruit, yogurt, soy, or nut or rice milk can also make a great protein addition to a diet. If your child has a tendency to crave sugars, eat too many carbohydrates, get sleepy after meals, or experience mood swings, protein intake should be increased to help stabilize blood sugar levels.

Fiber

Fiber is not a nutrient, yet it is an important dietary component. Fiber is found in fresh fruits, vegetables, legumes, whole grains, breads, and cereals. Fiber is essential to digestive health, keeping the digestive tract clean, lowering the risk of many gastrointestinal diseases, and binding toxins to be removed from the body.

Fiber helps to lower cardiovascular disease risk and binds cholesterol in the digestive tract so it is not absorbed. Fiber is not absorbed by the gut and is used to produce energy in the microflora of the intestines.

Vitamins

There are two types of vitamins: water-soluble and fat-soluble. Vitamins B and C are water-soluble so they must be taken in daily through the diet and can easily be lost or destroyed through contact with air, light, heat, or sunshine. Vitamins A, D, E, and K dissolve in fat and thus can be stored in the body's fatty tissue. These vitamins have the potential to be toxic in high doses.

Vitamin A

Vitamin A, a fat-soluble vitamin, is found in fish oils, milk products, liver, egg yolks, and carrots. Beta-carotene is another form of vitamin A found in green, yellow, and orange vegetables and fruits. Beta-carotene has the ability to be turned by the body into vitamin A. This was thought to be the main function of beta-carotene until recent research demonstrated that it is an antioxidant and immune nutrient with an important role in cancer prevention. Sources of beta-carotene include yams, carrots, winter squash, red bell pepper, broccoli, dark leafy greens, pink grapefruit, mangoes, apricots, and grapes. Lightly steaming the vegetables renders the beta-carotene more absorbable by the body than eating the vegetables raw. Juicing is an excellent way to get beta-carotene from raw vegetables. Vitamin A and beta-carotene improve immune function, increase resistance to infection, and aid in tissue repair. These nutrients are used in building healthy bones, skin, teeth, hair, eyes, blood cells, and mucous membranes throughout the body.

A deficiency of vitamin A increases the risk of infections in the eyes, nose, throat, and skin. Vitamin A is useful in treating acne, eczema, boils, and acute respiratory infections such as bronchitis, hypothyroidism, and measles.

Cod liver oil is an excellent way to get vitamin A as well as beneficial essential fatty acids.

B Complex Vitamins

The B complex is an important group of nutrients the body must acquire through the diet or from intestinal flora to transform food to energy, maintain a strong immune system, balance many of the body's hormones, and perform a number of other tasks. It is important to take B vitamins as a complex because each B vitamin has its own individual characteristics. Empty foods such as refined sugars and flours, alcohol, stress, and environmental pollution can deplete B vitamins. This makes it very important to acquire them daily in the food we eat.

Vitamin B1

Vitamin B1, or thiamine, is essential for a healthy nervous system and for breaking down food into energy. This nutrient is found in whole grains, oatmeal, millet, nuts, seeds, brewer's yeast, fish, peas, lentils, dried fruits, milk, eggs, and poultry. A B1 deficiency causes poor appetite, lack of energy, aggressive behavior, and lack of well-being. Vitamin B1 can be useful in treating fatigue, headache, irritability, and nerve pain.

Vitamin B2

Vitamin B2, or riboflavin, releases energy from foods and improves brain function, resistance to infection, red blood cell production, absorption of iron, and liver enzyme production. It is also an important cofactor for vitamin B6. Without vitamin B2, the body cannot use vitamin B6. Foods high in this vitamin include brewer's yeast, whole grains, cereals, milk, whole-wheat pasta, eggs, leafy greens, mushrooms, seafoods, nuts, and seeds. A lack of vitamin B2 commonly causes cracks or sores at the corners of the mouth and nose, poor appetite, light sensitivity, and skin rashes.

Vitamin B3

Vitamin B3, or niacin, reduces blood fats and forms enzymes necessary for carbohydrate metabolism. It also has a role in cholesterol metabolism. Signs of low vitamin B3 include poor appetite, sores at the corner of the mouth, diarrhea, skin problems, and moodiness. Foods high in this vitamin include meat, poultry, dairy, nuts, seeds, whole-grain breads, pastas, legumes, avocados, dried apricots, figs, mushrooms, leafy greens, peanuts, and cereals.

Vitamin B5

Vitamin B5, or pantothenic acid, is used in the metabolism of fats, amino acids, and carbohydrates and in the release of energy. The adrenal glands use it for normal function and production of the adrenal hormones. B5 is also used in immune function and wound healing. This vitamin can be very useful in treating conditions associated with stress. A B5 deficiency can lead to the development of allergies, pins-and-needles sensations, stomach cramps, tiredness, and restlessness. Vitamin B5 can be found in milk, eggs, leafy greens, brewer's yeast, nuts, wheat germ, mushrooms, whole grains, breads, cereals, legumes, and meats.

Vitamin B6

Vitamin B6, or pyridoxine, is needed for healthy brain function; production of red blood cells, antibodies, hormones, and enzymes; skin health; immune system health; and protein metabolism. It is useful in the treatment of asthma, skin rashes, heart disease, and inflammatory conditions. Cofactors for vitamin B6 metabolism are vitamin B2 and magnesium, both of which need to be present for the body to use B6. Foods rich in vitamin B6 include whole grains, nuts, bananas, egg yolks, fish, poultry, avocados, legumes and sprouted legumes, cabbage, corn, molasses, and pineapple.

Vitamin B12

Vitamin B12, or cyanocobalamin, is mainly found in meats, eggs, and dairy products and is almost entirely absent from plants. It is produced in small amounts by the intestinal flora. Foods fortified with vitamin B12 include cereals, some rice and soy milks, and yeast extracts. This is a crucial nutrient for the health of the nervous system, normal development of red blood cells, and iron metabolism. The body stores a small amount of vitamin B12, but chronic stress, poor stomach function, and vegan diets may lead to diminished B12 levels.

Folic Acid

This water-soluble vitamin is needed for healthy gums, skin, nervous system, and mucous membranes of the respiratory and gastrointestinal tracts. It is used along with vitamin B12 for cell division and red blood cell production. Folic acid is important in preventing heart disease, cancer, and birth defects. It is an important nutrient for a strong immune function, and it plays a role in antibody production.

Folic acid is found in most foods in some amounts except for fats, sugars, and alcohols. Foods that are especially high in folic acid are fresh leafy greens and green vegetables, wheat germ, whole grains, walnuts, almonds, bananas, broccoli, watercress, nettles, citrus fruits, dairy products, and eggs. Folic acid is not a stable vitamin and is lost easily with cooking, light, and storage. Thus, eating plenty of raw fruits and vegetables is important. Symptoms of deficiency include a sore tongue, cracks at the corners of the mouth, anemia, fatigue, depression, and susceptibility to infection. Supplement 200 micrograms, daily, for a child from 1 to 3 years old; 300 micrograms, for 4 to 6 years old; and 400 micrograms, for age 7 and older.

Vitamin C

Vitamin C, or ascorbic acid, has the widest range of use of any vitamin or mineral in both therapeutics and prevention. It also has been proved to be very safe and nontoxic. Some individuals will get loose bowels or stomach irritation from the acidity. Using a buffered vitamin C can eliminate this side effect. Vitamin C is an important antioxidant and immune-enhancing nutrient. It has strong antiviral activity, protects against radiation damage, and reduces heavy-metal toxicity in the body. It prevents free radical damage from toxins, drugs, smoke, pollution, and allergies. It is vital for healthy gums, skin, bones, muscles, blood vessels, and all other collagen tissue. Vitamin C enhances iron absorption and protects vitamins such as B_1, B_2, B_5, folic acid, and vitamins A and E from deteriorating in the body.

Foods high in vitamin C include all fresh fruits, vegetables, and leafy herbs. Especially high are citrus fruits, berries, broccoli, tomatoes, green peppers, cabbage, leafy greens, and potatoes. Vitamin C is an unstable vitamin that is diminished by light, heat, air, or storage. The diet should be able to provide an adequate amount of vitamin C if the child eats a good variety of fresh fruits and vegetables. If a child is unwell often; gets repeated earaches, colds, or runny noses; has allergies, hay fever, or asthma; or is easily bruised, vitamin C supplementation may be helpful. Children up to 3 years old can take 50 to 100 milligrams, daily; 3 to 5 years old, 250 milligrams, daily; 5 to 12 years old, 500 to 1,000 milligrams, daily.

Vitamin D

This fat-soluble vitamin is produced in our skin from sunlight and cholesterol. It aids in the absorption and utilization of calcium in the body and is essential for healthy bone and teeth formation and growth. Most children who get lots of fresh air and sunshine make plenty of vitamin D and store it in their bodies. Children who live in very overcast or smoggy areas may not produce as much and may benefit from foods high in the nutrient. Foods rich in vitamin D include fish, fish oils, dairy, eggs, and fortified cereals. Excessive levels of vitamin D can be toxic so prolonged supplementation is not recommended.

Vitamin E

This potent antioxidant nutrient is needed in the body for metabolism of essential fatty acids, red blood cell production, heart and blood vessel health, wound healing, and immune function. As an antioxidant, it prevents free radical damage in the blood vessels, heart, and nervous system. The best sources of vitamin E are wheat germ, cold-pressed vegetable oils, nuts, seeds, whole grains, eggs, avocados, butter, cheese, and seaweed.

Vitamin K

Vitamin K is vital for the production of blood-clotting factors, bone formation, and regulation of blood calcium levels. Some food sources of vitamin K include leafy greens, broccoli, seaweed, soybean oil, egg yolk, and garlic, but it is also produced by the beneficial microflora of the colon. When the colon is healthy, most of the vitamin K needed can be supplied. If the colon is low in beneficial microflora, such as after antibiotic therapy, vitamin K production will be affected. Including a good live-culture acidophilus yogurt in the diet or acidophilus capsules after antibiotic treatment can promote return of the healthy microflora.

Minerals

Many minerals find their way into our foods through the soils they are grown in. A diet high in good-quality organic fruits and vegetables is going to provide most of the needed minerals for your child. Mineral supplements are best absorbed from the digestive tract in a chelated form. There are varying degrees of absorbability, depending on the chelation substances, the highest absorbed forms being malate, citrate, fumarate, succinate, picolinate, and glycinate. Moderately well-absorbed are aspartate, sulfate, gluconate, and phosphate. Least absorbed and least expensive are carbonate and oxide. In the long run, the more absorbable types work out to be less expensive.

Calcium

Calcium is needed for healthy bones, skin, teeth, heart function, blood clotting, muscle function, nerve impulse function, and many other bodily functions. Dairy products are a rich source of calcium including yogurt, milk, cheese, and eggs. However, dairy products are also high in phosphorus and protein, which encourage excretion of calcium from the body. Many vegetables can be used to provide additional sources of calcium without using dairy products, including seaweeds, almonds, soy products, leafy greens, whole-wheat pasta, nuts, seeds, figs, prunes, apricots, molasses, and whole-grain breads.

If the diet is low in calcium-rich foods, supplement children one to twelve years old with 100 to 600 milligrams, daily, of a good chelated calcium with magnesium. Supplementation can ease growing pains, insomnia, restlessness, muscle cramps, allergies, and chronic infection.

Iron

This mineral is needed in the production of hemaglobin, the part of the red blood cell that delivers oxygen to all tissues of the body. Iron plays an important role in energy production, immune function, growth, and protein metabolism. Heme iron, one of the best forms of iron, is found in meats, poultry, and fish and seems to be the most readily absorbed food form. Plant sources of iron are many, but other substances that bind iron in the plants are present and make them less usable by the body. Eating a vitamin C–rich food with plant sources of iron will increase its absorbability, as will soaking grains for twenty-four hours and then cooking in fresh water. Plant sources rich in iron include leafy greens, green vegetables, dried fruits, whole grains, whole-wheat pasta, molasses, parsley, nettles, yellow dock, and soy.

Healthy infants have adequate iron stores for growth until they double their birth weight. This occurs at about four months in full-term babies. Babies from the age of six months to three years need a daily intake of 15 milligrams of iron. Breast milk has a highly bioavailable iron, which makes breast-feeding an asset during infancy. Most babies should receive some additional sources of iron at six months of age. Most iron is commonly provided through foods rich in iron and fortified cereals.

Children from one to three years old are at risk for iron deficiency anemia for several reasons. First, they have just finished a rapid growth period in their infancy, which uses large amounts of iron. Second, they are at an age where they continue to have high needs for iron. Finally, children at this age are often picky about the foods they eat, especially vegetables.

Magnesium

This mineral is needed for energy production from carbohydrates, protein metabolism, and burning of fat. It is needed for healthy bones, teeth, and muscle formation. Magnesium is required in enzyme production. It protects the cardiovascular and nervous systems and functions to enhance immunity. Magnesium is an important cofactor to many body processes, particularly insulin activity. It is depleted in the body by stress, exercise, and pollutants, making the body's need for this nutrient high. Most children do not get enough magnesium in their diets and are at risk of having insufficient tissue levels. Signs of low magnesium levels include muscle spasms, muscle twitches and tremors, tension, irritability, hyperactivity, insomnia, depression, weakness, and poor memory.

Food sources rich in magnesium include raw nuts, seeds, whole grains, legumes, leafy greens, fresh vegetable juices, dairy products, seafood, seaweed, millet, dried apricots, and soy products.

Potassium

Potassium works with sodium in the body to regulate the fluid balance throughout the tissues and organs. The ratio of potassium to sodium is higher in the muscles, organs, and soft tissues, while sodium is higher in the blood and intestinal fluids. This ratio determines acid/base regulation of the blood and body fluids and the function of nerve and muscle conduction. Often, the diet is higher in sodium intake than potassium, leading to a disturbance of the ratio between these two nutrients. Potassium is found in all fresh fruits, vegetables, and grains. Refining and processing of these foods, as with white flour or apple juice, remove the potassium. Other sources of potassium are nuts, dairy, soy beans, and seafood. Some signs of low potassium are insomnia, muscle cramps, fatigue, constipation, and bloating.

Phosphorus

This mineral is used with calcium for formation and health of the teeth and bones. It plays a role in heart, kidney, and nervous system function. It is also a cofactor in the body's metabolic functions. Phosphorus is present in many foods: milk, eggs, cereals, fruits, whole grains, nuts, seeds, vegetables, and fish.

Trace Minerals

Trace minerals are substances found in the body that are used in conjunction with other vitamins and minerals. They perform many subtle interactions in the body. The trace mineral content of the American diet is declining rapidly due to soil depletion, refining of foods, and poor eating habits. Sea vegetables are excellent sources of most trace minerals.

Zinc

The trace mineral zinc has many jobs in the body. As a component of many enzymes and enzymatic functions, it is required in protein metabolism, blood sugar metabolism, and the formation of RNA and DNA. It is one of the most important nutrients for immune function, hormonal function, and healthy bones, skin, and joints. Zinc aids in wound healing and in keeping the body's mucous membranes healthy. It is required for the sense of smell, taste, and adequate appetite. Cravings for sugar and carbohydrates can be due to low zinc levels. As an antioxidant, zinc helps to prevent free radical damage to the eyes, brain, prostate, and sperm.

Children who suffer from recurring ear infections, allergies, or respiratory infections have an increased need for zinc. Children living with smokers and exposed to secondary smoke will also be at risk for zinc deficiency. A simple taste test using a liquid zinc sulfate is an easy way to assess zinc levels. If one experiences little or no unpleasant taste, supplementation would be useful.

Foods high in zinc include shellfish, oysters, poultry, nuts, seeds, pumpkin seeds, egg yolks, ginger, split peas, fruits, asparagus, spinach, corn, and dairy products. Zinc is also found in many whole grains, yet it is bound with phytates that make it less absorbable. Soaking the grain for twelve hours and cooking it in fresh water may help to weaken the bonds.

Zinc deficiencies can contribute to loss of taste, slow growth, brittle hair and nails, acne, eczema, chronic infection, allergy, poor wound healing, delayed sexual development, poor appetite, poor digestion, abnormal behavior, dyslexia, and chemical hypersensitivity. It is also useful to supplement with zinc to decrease high levels of heavy metals such as lead, copper, and cadmium and to aid burn patients.

Chromium

This trace mineral is low in the average American diet, as it is lost in our food sources because of refining and processing.

Chromium helps the body use the hormone insulin more effectively and keeps the blood sugar balanced. It is vital for carbohydrate and fat metabolism and the production of energy. It enhances growth and protects the blood vessels from plaque buildup. Foods high in chromium include brewer's yeast, molasses, wheat germ, potato skins, oysters, nuts, whole grains, seafood, chicken, and fresh fruits and vegetables.

Selenium

Selenium is another essential trace mineral needed for optimal health and disease prevention. It is a strong antioxidant acting to quench free radicals, prevent tissue damage, inhibit inflammation, and remove toxic substances from the body. Selenium works with vitamin E to prevent tissue breakdown and protect from environmental chemical toxins. Foods rich in this mineral include brewer's yeast, wheat germ, garlic, eggs, whole grains, Swiss chard, mushrooms, cabbage, carrots, seaweed, meats, and seafood. Organically grown produce will be higher in this mineral than nonorganically grown. Supplement to remove heavy metals such as lead from the body or for suppressed immune systems.

Iodine

Iodine is vital to the thyroid gland for the production of thyroid hormones and function. The thyroid hormones are essential for the regulation of metabolism and physical/mental development. Iodine should be found in the soil and taken into the body through vegetables. Much of the soil vegetables are grown in is low in iodine due to the lack of organic fertilizers. Thus, our vegetables do not always supply iodine. Sea vegetables and seafoods are excellent sources of iodine as are organically grown garlic, onions, and parsley. Using seaweed powders in

soups, casseroles, and sauces can be a way to include sea vegetables in the diet. A teaspoon or so should add a little salty flavor to food without overpowering the taste. Iodized salt will also
add iodine to the diet.

Manganese

Manganese is another vitally important trace mineral in energy
production, healthy bone and cartilage formation, thyroid function, brain function, and nervous system health. Its antioxidant
effect protects against free radical damage and iron toxicity. Food
sources include leafy greens, nuts, seeds, dried figs, peaches,
dates, potatoes, bananas, whole grains, brewer's yeast, and eggs.
Manganese can quiet a histamine-related allergic response in the
immune system, as with hives or hayfever. Most multivita-
min/mineral supplements contain it.

Essential Fatty Acids:
The Key to a Strong Immune System

Modern research and clinical observation suggest that consumption of essential fatty acids (EFAs) is key to optimal health and
healthy development of the immune system throughout life.
Research has also demonstrated that EFAs reduce cholesterol levels in the growing years and have a protective effect against heart
disease later in life.

Since the body does not make its own EFAs and they must be
provided through the diet, an EFA deficiency is a real danger.
Moreover, EFAs are fragile and easily damaged by air, light, high
temperatures, and food processing. Therefore, if a child's diet is
high in processed refined foods and hydrogenated fats and she
avoids the foods that provide essential vitamins and minerals, she

is at risk for EFA deficiency. These crucial nutrients are most abundant in cold-water fish, dried legumes, and raw nuts and seeds.

Many of us know that there are good fats and bad fats. We are constantly hearing about the association between high levels of saturated fats and cholesterol and heart disease. Fatty acids, which are building blocks for fats, come in two forms: saturated and unsaturated. Saturated fatty acids make a fat that is solid and stiff at room temperature, such as margarine, hard cheese, and lard. The body needs some saturated fats, but all that is needed can be produced by the body. This means we don't actually need to provide any in the diet. Yet most of the fats consumed in the Western diet are saturated fats. Saturated fatty acids not only clog up the blood vessels but they interfere with the metabolism and use of EFAs in the body, leading to a compromise in the immune system.

Unsaturated fatty acids make a fat that is a liquid at room temperature. This includes most of the vegetable oils such as soy, sunflower, safflower, corn, olive, and canola. An important point to understand is that all EFAs are unsaturated fats, but not all unsaturated fats are EFAs. As with saturated fatty acids, the body can make all the nonessential, unsaturated fatty acids it needs without depending on dietary sources. A diet too high in nonessential, unsaturated fatty acids can also interfere with the metabolism and use of EFAs.

Unfortunately, many vegetable oils are subjected to a process called hydrogenation to prolong shelf life. This process actually converts unsaturated fatty acids to saturated fatty acids. Many processed foods such as crackers, chips, cookies, cereals, sauces, and so on are made with hydrogenated or partially hydrogenated vegetable oils. Margarine is made from hydrogenated vegetable oil, which makes it an antinutrient. Hydrogenated vegetable oils play havoc in the body, creating free radical damage, interrupt-

Role of EFAs in the Body

- Contribute to immune health and development
- Regulate activity of the white blood cells (macrophages, lymphocytes)
- Necessary in the production of prostaglandins
- Vital components of the cell membrane
- Vital components for building hormones
- Protect the body from cold
- Prevent allergy
- Necessary for cardiovascular health
- Promote a healthy nervous system and brain function

ing EFAs' metabolism and use, increasing cholesterol levels, and increasing inflammation. Heating or cooking with unsaturated fatty acids will destroy their beneficial action.

There are two groups of EFAs. Omega 6 oils comprise the first group and are found in the seeds of many plants, such as sunflower, safflower, corn, or evening primrose. Because of the trend to use vegetable oils in dressings and cooking, most children get adequate levels in their diet. However, they may not be able to use the oils efficiently if vitamin and mineral cofactors are unavailable.

The second group consists of omega 3 oils. This is the most deficient group of oils in the Western diet. Omega 3 oils are found mostly in fresh cold-water fish, such as salmon and cod. Cod liver oil is a great source of omega 3 oils. Omega 3 oils are found in flaxseeds and flaxseed oil along with wheat germ. The latter is very unstable and spoils rapidly so only freshly ground wheat germ should be used. The canning process depletes the amounts of omega 3 found in fish, as does the addition of vegetable oils, so fresh fish is the best source. Beans and legumes are excellent sources of both omega 3 and 6 oils and, if eaten regularly, can be excellent sources of EFAs.

Omega 3 and 6 oils are converted through an enzyme-regulated chemical reaction to other chemical forms called prostaglandins, which are active in many body processes. In order for the enzymes to regulate EFA metabolism, they depend on cofactors, vitamins, and minerals such as vitamin B6, C, E, zinc, magnesium, copper, and selenium. As long as the cofactors are present, EFAs can be converted into prostaglandins. Prostaglandins enhance immune protection, regulate white blood cell activity, and prevent allergic reaction. They play an important role in the disease process, and imbalances can lead to chronic disease. For example, a low dietary intake of EFAs combined with a high intake of saturated fatty acids will lead to an increased level of inflammation and inflammatory factors in the body, while a diet high in EFAs combined with a lower intake of saturated fatty acids will lead to a low level of inflammation and a higher level of anti-inflammatory factors. Hence, one diet will support a diseased state and the other will prevent or decrease the same condition, as with asthma, allergy, or eczema.

Signs of EFA Deficiency: How Can I Tell if My Child Is Low?

Because EFAs are used in the makeup of every body cell membrane, we can see signs of deficiency in many places, including hair, skin, and nails. Skin signs of low EFAs include dry, scaly, bumpy skin. Often the backs of the arms and legs will get bumpy and rough. Skin, as well as the hair, will look dull with no luster or shine. Fingernails can be brittle or dry and may crack easily.

A child who has chronic, repeated congestion; runny nose; earache; cough; or wounds that are slow to heal is often in need of EFAs. Allergy reactions of all kinds—hay fever, asthma, skin rash, and digestive problems—all respond to EFA supplementation.

How Can I Get Enough EFAs into My Child?

Diet is the smartest way to provide EFAs to a child. A diet that is rich in raw nuts, nut butters, seeds, fish, and beans and low in hydrogenated or saturated fats will probably provide adequate amounts for a healthy child. If the child suffers from allergy, skin rash, chronic colds, earaches, asthma, or low immune resistance, or does not eat foods high in EFAs, EFA-rich food oils may be the easiest and most practical approach to take. Oils high in EFAs can be added to foods such as dips, salad dressings, cereals, or other food recipes. Supplementation with oils in a gel cap form are easiest for the older child to chew or swallow.

Flaxseed Oil

Flaxseed oil is usually found in the refrigerator section of the natural food store or co-op. It is a mix of omega 3 and 6 fatty acids, the majority being omega 3. Select a brand that is unrefined, made with no extra heat, and labeled with the date of processing. Flax oil will store in the refrigerator for four months and in the freezer for up to eight months from the date of processing. If flaxseed oil tastes bitter rather than mildly sweet, it is rancid and should not be used. Flaxseed oil can be given directly from a teaspoon, which some children don't mind, or in food preparation.

- As a salad dressing, use half-and-half with olive oil.
- Add to cooked vegetables, cereal, or pasta instead of butter.

- For a healthy, good-tasting butter alternative, combine and blend ½ cup each flaxseed oil and sweet butter.
- Add to vegetable dips, spreads, shakes, and smoothies.

For additional recipes, see pages 64–71. Flaxseed oil should never be heated, but it can be added to warm foods.

Fish Oils and Cod Liver Oil

These are available in gel cap form and may be useful in treating EFA-deficiency conditions. Cod liver oil is available in flavored liquid form for young children who cannot chew or swallow the gel caps. Use ½ to 1 teaspoon, daily.

Evening Primrose Oil

This oil is rich in omega 6 fatty acids. In some cases, these EFAs are needed in higher levels than the omega 3s. Treatment of conditions such as hyperactivity and allergies should include omega 6 oils. Other sources of omega 6 are borage seed oil and black currant seed oil. Dosage is 1 to 2, 500 milligram capsules, daily.

GUIDELINES AND TIPS FOR HEALTHY EATING

Dairy

Milk and other dairy products often stimulate allergies and are best avoided by most children. In an allergic child, the body responds to the antigen from the milk as though it were a foreign microbial invader. This taxes the immune system, making it less able to respond with its full force when a truly dangerous bacteria or virus appears. If your child has allergic tendencies of any kind, take milk and other dairy products off the menu. Dairy products have other problems as well. They often stimulate mucous production in the respiratory system, adding to congestion and thickening secretions and putting the child at risk for frequent colds, earaches, and a perpetual stuffy nose.

The saturated fats in dairy products also work against the beneficial fatty acids in the child's diet, which are so essential to optimal health.

Milk Substitutes

The following can be used on top of cereal, in baking, or whenever milk is called for in any recipe: rice milk (sometimes called amasake), soy milk, almond (or other nut) milk, goat's milk, sheep's milk, or diluted fruit juice (except for orange).

Cheeses

Some natural hard cheeses can be kept in the diet for occasional use. However, avoid yellow cheeses (they contain dyes) and highly processed cheeses. Choose white hard cheese; raw milk cheese is the best choice because of the positive amounts of live active cultures. Many delicious soy cheeses are on the market today.

Butter

Use sweet butter instead of margarine or other hydrogenated products that can create free radicals in the body and thus work against the immune system. Keep butter use to a minimum, or try the following excellent alternative.

Better Butter Recipe

Mix ½ cup flaxseed oil with ½ cup softened sweet butter. Blend well and refrigerate. Makes a healthy, delicious spread for bread or to top vegetables. Do not heat or use for cooking.

Other oils—such as flaxseed, sunflower, sesame, or walnut— that are rich in the beneficial omega 3 and omega 6 oils can add flavor and nutrients to cooked or raw foods. Try flaxseed oil over cooked rice, or olive oil seasoned with garlic or a few herbs on toasted bread. Any of these oils or nutritional yeast plus a sprinkling of herbs make a great topping for freshly popped popcorn. These oils should not be heated, although they can be placed atop hot foods. Use olive or canola oils for cooking.

Yogurt

Yogurt is a good food as long as it contains live bacterial cultures. Low-fat yogurt is best because of its perfect balance of protein to carbohydrate to fat. One cup of low-fat yogurt is a complete and adequate protein snack, as long as it is plain (or with unsweetened fruit) and has live active cultures. Yogurt can be used with cereal, in smoothie drinks, or as a snack with fresh fruit.

Eggs

Eggs are good sources of protein and can be added to any meal. However, they should not be introduced into a baby's diet before fifteen months of age because the baby may have trouble digesting the egg protein (primarily in the egg white) before that time. Introduce the yolk first. Avoid giving eggs to highly allergic children, especially those with severe eczema or severe asthma.

Grains

Whole grains provide many vitamins and minerals as well as fiber. Grains may be eaten in the whole form, as in oatmeal or brown rice, or in pasta, breads, crackers, cereals, and flours. Avoid white, enriched, processed, and refined flour products, as these products have little nutritional value and also contain excess sugar, salt, and preservatives. Choose whole-grain cereals, crackers, breads, and pasta. Whole grains still have all their parts including the bran and the germ. These include brown rice, basmati rice, millet, buckwheat, whole oats (groats), quinoa, amaranth, whole-wheat flours, wheatberries, and barley. Grains are rich in fiber, B vitamins, and other essential nutrients.

Proteins

Proteins are a very important part of the daily diet and should be included at every meal. At breakfast, the milks that you use with your cereals (cow, rice, soy, almond, or yogurt) can be the protein source. Other protein sources are cheeses, meats, fish, nuts, seeds, nut butters, tofu, tempeh burgers, and legumes such as lentils and chick peas. Eating cold-water fish, such as cod, halibut, salmon, and tuna, is recommended several times per week. Sea vegetables included in soup stocks and stews are also great sources of protein and iron.

Limit the amount of red meat in your child's diet. Red meat is difficult to digest and directly enters into the inflammatory cascade, perpetuating inflammation reactions in the immune system. Eat only small amounts of red meat and opt instead for fish and poultry. Remember that legumes are also excellent protein sources, but sometimes they are difficult to digest. If this is the case, give digestive enzymes with a bean meal. Use beans in combination with whole grains for an inexpensive but complete protein/carbohydrate meal such as black beans and rice. Tofu, tempeh, and other soy products are good sources of vegetable protein, as is texturized vegetable protein.

Fruits

Fruits are generally a good addition to the diet. They are rich in fiber, pectins, and vitamins and minerals. However, fruit should be eaten in moderation, and some should be avoided altogether. Eating too many fruits or drinking large amounts of fruit juice leads to too much simple sugar (fructose) in your child's diet, which can be more harmful than helpful. Oranges are very allergenic and can exacerbate gastrointestinal symptoms, skin symptoms, mental/emotional symptoms, or fatigue. Do not give your child oranges or orange juice daily. Bananas are also difficult to digest and are very high in fruit sugars. They are also highly allergenic and often cause infantile eczema. Berries and grapes, on the other hand, offer a rich source of bioflavonoids and make an excellent addition to most children's diets.

Nuts and Seeds

Nuts and seeds are great sources of protein and healthy fats. Some nut butters are excellent food sources, while others are highly allergenic. Nuts and seeds are best eaten raw or roasted by you at home. Commercially roasted nuts often contain rancid oils.

Avoid or limit peanuts and peanut butters. They are highly allergenic and can cause a number of symptoms that range from digestive problems to immune system depression. Use almond, cashew, hazelnut, sesame butter (tahini), or sunflower seed butter instead of peanut butter. Store raw nuts and nut butters in the refrigerator.

HEALTHY RECIPES

Immune Support Breakfast*

The modern American diet, which is high in refined carbohydrates, wreaks havoc with the body's digestive and elimination systems. By strengthening the body's eliminative function, the functioning of the immune system is also greatly enhanced. The following recipe is not designed to be hypoallergenic and must be modified for your child's personal dietary profile. It must also be used 2 to 4 times a week over a period of 2 months for the effects to be noticeable. People who use it regularly notice fewer allergic responses.

4 cups rolled grains (such as oats or barley)
2 cups oat bran
1 cup dried fruit
1 cup sunflower seeds, ground
1 cup raw, unsalted nuts, chopped
1 cup lecithin granules
1 cup flaxseed, ground

Mix all ingredients well and store in refrigerator. For each serving, soak ½ cup dry mixture at least 30 minutes (overnight is okay) in soy milk, nut milk, rice milk, diluted fruit juice, or water. To increase protein value, eat with yogurt or tofu.

*Recipe developed by Bruce Milliman, N.D.

Fruit Smoothie

½ banana
2 ice cubes
1 cup juice (such as apple, grape, pear, berry, or pineapple)

1 Tbs. plain yogurt with live cultures
1 Tbs. flaxseed oil

Add all ingredients together in a blender and mix. Protein powder, fresh or frozen berries, or other fruits may also be added. Makes a great breakfast drink.

**Dr. Bill Mitchell's Ginger Soup
(An immune system booster)**
6 cups water
3 Tbs. gingerroot, chopped
10 scallions, chopped
1 brick tofu, cubed
3 cups bean sprouts
3 Tbs. tamari
½ tsp. red pepper
1 tsp. paprika
1 head garlic, peeled and chopped
Juice of 1 lemon

Coat inside of a wok or pan with olive oil. Add all ingredients and simmer for 15 to 20 minutes.

Potassium Broth
Organic vegetables are the best not only because they are free of toxic pesticides but they contain more nutrients than nonorganic vegetables.

½-inch outer peelings, including skins, of 3 potatoes
Bunch fresh parsley, chopped
3 scrubbed, unpeeled carrots, cut into rounds
Handful beet greens, chopped
2 medium onions, chopped

5 cloves garlic, crushed
Other green leafy vegetables, chopped
2 quarts water

Wash and prepare vegetables. Simmer in water in large covered pot for 30 to 40 minutes. Strain. Excess broth may be stored in refrigerator for up to 2 days.

Dill Salad Dressing

This dressing is great on salads, grains, vegetables, or fish.

⅓ cup fresh dill, minced
¼ cup cider vinegar or lemon juice
1 ½ Tbs. Dijon mustard
½ tsp. honey or rice syrup
½ cup flaxseed oil

In a bowl or blender mix everything except the flaxseed oil. Slowly pour in the flaxseed oil while blending or whisking vigorously, until the dressing is thick and smooth. Keep extra dressing refrigerated in a dark bottle for later use.

Ginger Salad Dressing

3 Tbs. flaxseed oil
1–2 Tbs. fresh lemon juice
1 tsp. gingerroot, grated
1 clove garlic, minced

Whisk the ingredients together and store in the refrigerator in a dark bottle.

Tamari Salad Dressing

¼ cup flaxseed oil
2–3 tsps. tamari

2–3 tsps. apple cider vinegar
1–3 cloves garlic, minced

Adjust the proportions to taste. To vary the flavor, add a few pinches of one or more of the following: onion powder, basil, oregano, or curry powder.

Almond Milk
½ cup almonds
2 cups water

Put the almonds into a jar, cover with water, and soak 12 to 24 hours. Drain off the water and thoroughly rinse the nuts. Blanch the almonds in boiling water for 30 seconds. Squeeze the almonds between the fingertips to remove the skins. Blend the almonds and ½ cup of water until smooth, about 1 minute. While the blender is running, slowly add the remaining ½ cup of water and continue to blend for 1 more minute. Strain, if desired. This may be kept covered and refrigerated for 2 to 3 days.

Almond Pesto Rice Salad
2 cups brown basmati rice
3 ½ cups water
¾ cup raw almonds
½ bunch of parsley
½ bunch fresh basil
2 cloves garlic
3 Tbs. lemon juice
3 Tbs. olive oil
½ cucumber, cut in quarter moons

Bring the rice and water to a boil, turn down the heat, and simmer for 45 minutes. Add the remaining ingredients, reserving the cucumber, to a blender and puree. Put the cooked rice in a bowl to cool. While still warm add the pesto sauce and continue to cool. Add cucumber to the rice when cool. Adjust seasoning to taste.

Tofu Spread
1 cup firm tofu, mashed
1 clove garlic, crushed
1 Tbs. each: carrot, celery, and onion, grated
1 tsp. parsley, chives, or basil, chopped

Mash all ingredients together in a bowl. Use a blender to puree if a smoother consistency is desired.

Wild Food Recipes

Sorrel Soup
2 cups garden sorrel or French sorrel, chopped
1 small onion, chopped
2 cloves garlic, chopped
2 medium potatoes, chopped
1 quart vegetable stock
1 Tbs. butter
Nutmeg to taste

Steam sorrel lightly and sauté with garlic, onions, butter, and nutmeg. Add the potatoes and stock and cook until the potatoes are soft. Puree in blender. Serve with a teaspoon of yogurt on top. May also be made with lovage, nettles, spinach, or chard.

Pumpkin Flower Fritters
1 egg, separated
1 Tbs. milk

1 Tbs. olive oil
4 Tbs. flour
1/4 tsp. savory or marjoram
Pumpkin flowers

Beat egg yolk, milk, and oil; sift in flour and let stand for 30 minutes. Beat egg white until stiff; fold into flour mixture and add savory or marjoram. Dip pumpkin flowers into the batter and fry in olive oil until brown. May also use elder flowers.

Rosehip Sauce
2 cups rosehips
2 cups water
1 cup sugar

Put water and sugar in a pan and boil until the sugar has melted; slice hips in half and add to sugar mixture; cook gently for 1 hour. Strain through a sieve and cool.

Basil Butter
3 basil leaves, finely chopped
1 lemon balm leaf, finely chopped
1/2 lb. soft butter

With a wooden spoon mix the leaves into the butter until creamy.

Burdock Pickles
Wash and slice burdock root to desired size, steam, and pack into pint-size canning jar. Save steaming liquid.

Mix together:
1/2 head garlic
1 slice of gingerroot

⅓ cup steaming liquid
⅓ cup tamari
⅓ cup Chinese vinegar or rice vinegar

Pour over the burdock root and seal jar. Let stand for 24 hours.

Nettle Loaf
3 cups steamed nettles, pureed
2 Tbs. celery, chopped
2 Tbs. onion, chopped
2 Tbs. butter, melted
2½ cups cooked brown rice
3 eggs, beaten

Combine all ingredients and pour into a well-greased loaf pan. Bake at 350° F for 30 minutes. Serve with tahini sauce (recipe follows) or pesto sauce.

Tahini Sauce
¼ cup raw tahini
¼ cup warm water
1 Tbs. soy sauce
1 tsp. lemon juice

Mix well with whisk and serve.

Soup of Potherbs
This is a wonderful soup to make in the spring when the herbs are young and tender. The herbs help cleanse the body and revive it for spring.

½ cup each: fresh washed nettles, lovage, and French
   sorrel, chopped

1 small onion, diced
2 cloves garlic, chopped
1 Tbs. olive oil
Half a lemon, juiced
3 cups water
1 vegetable boullion cube

Sauté the onion and garlic in the olive oil until soft. Steam the greens and puree with a little of the steaming juice. Heat water and dissolve boullion. Add all other ingredients and simmer gently for 20 minutes.

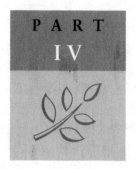

Common
Childhood Illnesses

See Part VI for instructions on how to make the recommended herbal preparations.

ASTHMA

Asthma is a lung disease characterized by inflammation of the bronchial tree, obstruction of the airways, spasms of the smooth muscles of the bronchial tree, and an accumulation of thick mucus in the lungs. This results in hyperinflation of the lungs, trapping the air and stopping the child from exhaling sufficiently. Shortness of breath, cough, a sensation of air hunger, and wheezing are symptomatic; it is harder for a child to breathe out than to breathe in. The wheezing is a high-pitched whistling sound more prominent on exhalation than on inhalation (in contrast to croup). Generally, a child who has asthma will have a chronic underlying condition with acute episodes of bronchospasm.

When not experiencing the acute attacks, the child may simply have mild wheezing or a chronic irritating cough.

An acute asthma attack may last for minutes, hours, or days. During an attack several factors combine to make breathing difficult. The muscles constrict and narrow the air passages; the mucous membranes swell and thicken, reducing the air passages; and the mucous secretions become thick, also blocking the airways. The air hunger and inability to exhale and inhale sufficiently often lead to panic and fear during the attack, which tend to make things worse. Asthma attacks are more likely to occur at night but often occur after either physical or emotional stress. The physical stress can be exercise, an allergenic food, exposure to irritating substances, or infectious/inflammatory processes. The emotional stress can come from a variety of stimuli, not the least of which may be the memory of a previous acute attack.

A variety of triggers alone or in combination may initiate the onset of the attack. In addition to resolving an acute attack, the chronic asthmatic condition will also need to be addressed in a more long-term approach. Common causes of asthma include:

Allergies: Substances such as dust, pollen, animal dander, mold, and many foods can cause an allergic reaction that provokes an attack. There is often a family history of atopic conditions such as asthma, eczema, and hay fever.

Infections: Respiratory infections (bronchitis, cough, colds, flu) of the bronchial tree can cause irritation and inflammation, leading to bronchial constriction. Bronchitic asthma is most commonly seen in children between the ages of two and six years old. In addition to the usual symptoms of an asthma attack, accompanying symptoms include fever and dry cough.

Irritants: Airborne substances can irritate the airways and set off an attack. Common offenders are smoke, smog, chemicals, perfumes, cleaning products, cold air, and sawdust.

Emotional factors: Stressful situations, anxiety, nervousness, insecurity, or fear can all trigger an attack. A child might suffer an attack in a certain surrounding, when the family is disrupted, after a separation from a parent, or in response to a parent who is overly protective. The fact that the child has asthma and has experienced an acute attack is in itself an anxiety-producing thought. This factor often compounds the situation during an attack.

Family history: There may be an inherent disposition toward asthma in the child who has a relative or sibling who also suffers from asthma, eczema, or hay fever.

Digestive disturbances: Maldigestion and overeating may lead to an asthmatic attack by irritating the nervous tissue in the stomach, causing a reflex action through the nerve to the bronchial tree, resulting in bronchospasms. Additional factors to investigate include "leaky gut" syndrome or liver congestion; imbalances in digestive microflora, hydrochloric acid, or other digestive enzymes; or poor elimination of waste and toxins in the body, chronic constipation, and the overgrowth of fungus or parasites in the bowel.

Increased toxin load: An increased load of environmental toxins, such as food additives and colorings or pesticides, may also contribute to the condition.

When working to overcome the asthmatic condition, it is important to focus on the general vitality, wellness, and constitution of the child; to address all underlying factors; to minimize exposure to all irritants even if not positively identified as triggers; and to improve the functions and health of the immune, digestive, and respiratory systems. Treatment of the asthmatic condition can take several months to a few years.

Treatments

Dietary Guidelines

- Avoid high-allergen foods such as eggs, fish, shellfish, nuts, and peanuts, which usually cause an immediate reaction. Milk, chocolate, wheat, citrus, tomatoes, or food colorings and additives usually cause a more delayed onset reaction. Bananas might also be a problem.
- Avoid food additives such as azo dyes (tartrazine, sunset yellow, coccine) and non-azo dyes such as sodium benzoate, sulphur dioxide, and sulfites. Tartrazine is in many processed foods, vitamins, and some drugs. Sulphites are found in salad dressings, potato products, and avocado dip.
- A low intake of animal products such as meats, eggs, and dairy products can be helpful.
- Increase whole grains, fresh vegetables, fruits, and sesame seeds.
- Avoid processed and refined foods such as white-flour products, margarine, and hydrogenated oils.
- Use fresh, raw oils such as olive, flaxseed, sunflower, and sesame on salads, in dips and spreads, or in smoothies. Do not cook with these oils. Cook with olive or canola oil only.
- Give herbal teas or punches to build up the immune, digestive, detoxification, and respiratory systems of the body. Combine several of the tonic herbs such as astragalus root, calendula, cleavers, dandelion, hyssop, nettles, oats, red clover, ribwort, and yarrow flowers. Japanese green tea is

very high in flavonoids, which help to stabilize the mast cells and reduce inflammation. This may be taken alone or mixed with mint or anise to flavor. Drink 2 to 3 cups daily.

Vitamins and Minerals

Antioxidants such as beta-carotene, selenium, zinc, and vitamins E and C will help stabilize the chemical responses that trigger the attack and improve fatty acid metabolism. (See Essential Nutrients, page 39.)

The essential fatty acids gamma-linolenic acid and eicosapenanoic acid are particularly useful in blocking the chemicals that might trigger the bronchospasm. (See Essential Fatty Acids, page 54.)

The bioflavonoids, particularly quercetin, can help to stabilize histamine-releasing cell membranes, blocking the chemical inflammatory reaction. Give 300 milligrams, 3 times a day, together with vitamin C. This combination is available in one capsule at many health food stores. Magnesium is necessary for smooth muscle relaxation and may be useful in improving asthmatic breathing. Taking magnesium and vitamin C before exercise can help prevent the onset of an exercise-induced attack.

Treatments for Acute Asthma

In acute asthmatic attacks, the child must be assessed for the degree of emergency. If the attack is severe or does not respond to home treatments, call your doctor, 911, or seek emergency room treatment. Less severe or mild attacks can be managed with some of the following:

- Give a tincture made from ½ ounce each: lobelia, cramp-bark, ephedra, and licorice combined with ½ teaspoon of cayenne tincture. Use ½ teaspoon of the mix in a little warm water every 15 minutes. If the child does not respond after 2 to 3 hours of treatment, call the doctor.

- Use herbal inhalants of aromatic essential oils such as eucalyptus, lavender, peppermint, and yarrow as a steam, in a lukewarm bath, or apply with warm compresses to the chest and back.
- Sometimes cold compresses applied to the back of the neck and head help.
- Chest rubs made from relaxing and antispasmodic herbs will act to release the bronchospasm and make breathing easier. Try a mix of ½ ounce each of lobelia oil and cramp-bark tincture, ¼ ounce of cayenne oil, and 10 drops each of lavender and thyme essential oils.
- Cranberry is an effective antispasmodic and thins the mucus. Use 1 cup of fresh or frozen cranberries crushed with 1 cup of warm water. If necessary, sweeten this very sour mixture with an equal amount of apple juice. Drink freely.

Treatments for Chronic Asthma

Many herbs can address some of the underlying factors that predispose the child to asthma. Use herbs to strengthen and support the immune system, digestion, and lungs.

Lung herbs such as mullein, licorice, marshmallow root, and ribwort will help to reduce irritation and tone the membranes. Herbs such as hyssop, thyme, aniseed, and elecampane will relax the lungs and help to expel the mucus.

Use relaxing and calming herbs when emotional stress or anxiety is part of the picture. Think of chamomile, catnip, lemon balm, linden flower, passionflower, skullcap, and valerian.

Encourage fresh air and exercise to strengthen the lungs. Singing, blowing up balloons, and using abdominal breathing exercises can all be helpful.

ATHLETE'S FOOT (RINGWORM)

Ringworm is a fungal infection of the skin. It spreads by direct contact with an infected person or animal, or from contaminated objects such as combs, pillows, towels, clothing, bathroom floors, showers, and swimming pools. Different fungi prefer different areas of the body. Ringworm on the scalp appears as a scaly, oval dry patch with poor hair growth and broken hairs. Ringworm of the body appears as a round or oval red ring moving outward with healing in the center. Ringworm of the groin appears as a red-brown, scaly rash with well-defined margins that spread. Ringworm of the feet, commonly known as athlete's foot, affects the feet, toes, and ankles. Athlete's foot can cause intense itching and cracking of the toes and feet.

Treatments

Internal

Use herbs and supplements to boost the immune system. Limit junk foods, increase fiber, and provide adequate protein. (See Part III.) Herbal treatments can include herbal antifungals, alteratives, and circulatory stimulants. Try a mix of equal amounts of echinacea, usnea, calendula, licorice, and peppermint. Use this internally over several months combined with topical treatment to the area. If using a tea, drink ½ cup, 2 times a day; for a tincture, the dosage is ¼ teaspoon, 2 times a day.

Topical

A combination of several topical treatments can be effective, such as a footbath each evening with daytime use of a cream or oil.

- Herbal decoctions and infusions can be used to soak the feet or to apply as a wash. Bathe the area for 20 minutes, making sure to dry well, and apply an herbal powder to the area afterward. Choose herbs such as calendula, sage, echinacea, myrrh, witch hazel, or gentian.
- Herbal powders keep the area dry and free of moisture and deliver medical activity. Use a mix of powdered goldenseal, slippery elm, lavender, witch hazel, and bentonite. Apply several times a day and after bathing.
- Essential oils of thyme, tea tree, lavender, oregano, thuja, and rosemary can be applied to the lesions several times a day. Oils can be applied undiluted or diluted lightly if the child's skin is sensitive. Dilute 5 drops of essential oil with 2 to 3 drops of olive or sweet almond oil.
- An herbal liniment made of a combination of tinctures can be applied 3 to 4 times, daily. Mix equal parts of 2 or 3 of these tinctures: myrrh, calendula, oregano, thuja, greater celandine, sage, echinacea, usnea, or spilanthes.
- Iodine washes or applications can also be helpful.

BED-WETTING

Many children cannot remain dry for an entire night before the age of five. About 10 percent of all children over the age of five are bed-wetters. Underlying causes for bed-wetting include bladder infection, structural abnormality of the urinary tract, food allergy, nerve compression in the spinal cord, emotional factors, or diabetes.

Treatments

It is important to find out what the cause of the bed-wetting is. Your doctor can help you rule out infection with a few simple lab tests. Check for food allergies by eliminating the more common allergens from the diet. (See Food Allergy, page 31.) Restrict fluid intake at night but not as a punishment. Try not to overreact, shame the child, or get angry, as this will only worsen the situation. Try using a reward system for success such as a gold star or special sticker and a neutral response for "accidents."

BLISTERS

A blister is an accumulation of clear fluid between the layers of the skin. It may be caused by heat or chemical burns, rubbing and friction, allergy to bug bites, and bacterial or viral infections. A blister can range in size from that of a pinhead to several inches.

Treatments

- Do not break open the blister; cover and protect with gauze. If it does open, wash with vulnerary herbs like calendula, comfrey, yarrow, or a mild calendula soap, and apply a sterile bandage.
- Herbal compresses of astringent herbs, such as witch hazel, white oak bark, raspberry, or rosemary, can increase the movement of the fluid out of the blister and allow the skin to heal.

- If the blister becomes infected, it should be opened and soaked in Epsom salts (6 ounces salts to 1 pint water) or antiseptic herbs such as goldenseal, echinacea, tea tree, yarrow, or hyssop. Use an herbal salve to cover the new tender skin under the blistered skin.
- Use a poultice of black tea bags soaked in lukewarm water and apply to the blister for 15 minutes, 3 times a day. This will help to dry the fluid.
- Try compresses of yarrow and witch hazel tea to dry the fluid and avoid infection.

Elder Flowers Compress
1 Tbs. elder flowers
1 tsp. each: calendula flowers, raspberry leaf, and plantain

Use 1 pint of boiling water and make a strong tea. Let cool. Soak a washcloth in the cooled tea and apply to blistered area.

BOILS

Boils, also known as furuncles, are localized infections beneath the skin resulting from infection by the bacteria, staphylococcus. The boils are red and painful and form a pus-filled center that drains through the skin. They most often occur on the neck, face, chest, or buttocks. Boils found on the eyelids are called styes, small superficial boils on the skin are called pimples, and collections of pus in other parts of the body, such as the muscles, bones, or internal organs, are known as abscesses. When boils occur repeatedly and in many places, the condition is called furunculosis.

Staphylococcus bacteria are commonly found in the nose, throat, and skin as part of the microflora we live with. It is not usually a disease-producing microbe unless the immune system and the body's resistance are being stressed. They are thought to enter the body superficially from a break in the skin, an abrasion, or a rash. Staphylococcus also causes the skin condition impetigo.

Treatments

When treating a boil, I like to approach it both internally and externally. For inside the body, I would use herbs to support the immune system (echinacea, usnea, licorice) and the elimination system, especially the skin (burdock, dandelion, calendula, cleavers) plus acidophilus capsules. For outside the body, I would use hot soaks, compresses, poultices, and salves. Boils respond to frequent soaks with Epsom salts. Use 1 cup salts to 1 quart water. When the boil comes to a head and drains, clean it with calendula soap and use a little herbal salve. Some boils may not come to a head and may require lancing by a doctor.

If outbreaks of boils are frequent, strengthening the immune system and detoxifying the liver and bowel are essential steps to resolve the problem. Consider using teas and herbal punches made from nettles, red clover, dandelion leaf and root, calendula, echinacea, burdock, and fennel.

Immune and Skin Tea
Mix ½ ounce of each of the following herbs in a jar: cleavers, calendula flowers, red clover blossoms, licorice root, and nettles. Use 1 teaspoon of this mixture per cup of boiling water. Drink 2 to 3 times a day.

It is also important to make sure the diet is free from refined sugars, processed foods, preservatives, and poor-quality fats, and is high in fresh vegetables, fruits, whole foods, and lots of good-quality drinking water.

Hot soaks and compresses of herbal infusions and decoctions made from astringent herbs like myrrh, white oak bark, witch hazel bark, goldenseal root, or burdock root, applied 3 times a day, will help to drain the pus and act as an antiseptic.

Aromatic Drawing Bath or Soak

Mix 2 cups Epsom salts with 3 drops of essential oils of lavender and tea tree. Add essential oils, 2 to 3 drops at a time, mixing the salts well each time. Use 1 cup salts to a quart of water for soaking, or, if using as a full body bath, use 1 to 2 cups.

Drawing Poultices

Make a poultice from 1 tablespoon grated white potato and ½ teaspoon of slippery elm powder. Apply to boil and hold in place with a gauze pad for several hours.

Make a poultice from equal parts of goldenseal powder, slippery elm powder, marshmallow root powder, and bentonite. Mix a small amount of the powdered herbal mixture with enough water to make a paste, apply to the boil, and let dry. Repeat several times a day.

Herbal Soak or Wash

1 Tbs. each: comfrey leaf, yarrow flowers, calendula flowers, and raspberry leaf.
1 tsp. each: burdock root and echinacea root

Add the roots to 1 quart cold water, bring to a boil, cover, and simmer for 15 minutes. Take off the heat and stir in the rest of the herbs, cover, and steep for 15 minutes. Strain and use as hot as is tolerated as a soak or on a compress for 15 minutes, 4 to 5 times a day.

BRONCHITIS

Bronchitis is an inflammation of the mucous membranes lining the bronchial tubes of the respiratory system. Acute bronchitis is most commonly caused by a viral infection, but bacterial and fungal infections can also lead to bronchitis. Bronchitis is characterized by a dry, hacking cough; a low-grade fever of 100°F to 101°F (but sometimes no fever); tightness and pain of the chest; loss of appetite; and a general feeling of malaise. Cold symptoms may also be present. The cough starts to loosen after a few days, becoming more productive in expelling the mucus and phlegm. Sometimes a rattling sound can be heard with breathing. The illness usually lasts seven to ten days.

Chronic bronchitis can occur when a child gets frequent, acute episodes or when he or she is compromised by allergies, food intolerances, asthma, or a weakened immune system. Look at the child's health and lifestyle picture and address these in your treatments. (See Part II, Working with the Young Immune System, starting on page 19.) Chronic bronchitis causes a cough, yellow-white phlegm, and general lethargy. It can be aggravated by temperature changes, cold weather, and molds.

Treatments

- When treating chronic bronchitis use treatments to strengthen the immune system and the respiratory system. Give treatments to deal with allergies and chronic inflammation. The lung-strengthening herbs are horsetail, mullein, ribwort, and slippery elm.

- When treating acute bronchitis put together a formula of herbs that stimulates the immune response (echinacea, osha root, usnea, or wild indigo); acts as a respiratory antiseptic (garlic, hyssop, thyme, or yarrow); acts as an expectorant to loosen the cough and bring up the mucus (thyme, elecampane, or mullein); and acts as an antispasmodic to keep the cough from being too spastic (catnip, crampbark, lemon balm, or skullcap). Give the formula as a hot tea with a dash of ginger added several times a day or use in tincture form, ½ to 1 teaspoon, 3 to 4 times a day.
- If there is a fever give chamomile, elder flowers, linden flowers or meadowsweet to help the body keep the fever productive in fighting the infection. (See Fever, page 127.)
- Give a syrup to loosen the cough, quiet the spasms, and start the bronchial secretions flowing in the first stage of the cough. Here is a good combination. Combine equal parts of thyme, licorice, and white pine bark and ½ parts each: lobelia, cinnamon, and ginger. (See Making Herbal Preparations, starting on page 259, for the procedure.) When the cough has turned loose and productive, use herbs to support it such as aniseed, elecampane, mullein, and licorice. (See Cough, page 105.)
- Chest rubs are useful in increasing circulation and in warming and relaxing the chest and respiratory muscles. They are best applied topically before bed or napping. Then cover the chest with a cotton T-shirt. Rubs usually contain aromatic herbs such as eucalyptus, hyssop, thyme, peppermint, camphor, or rosemary, which are very volatile and therefore penetrate the skin easily, stimulate blood flow, relax the muscles, and deliver medication to the local area. They can be especially effective with spastic, tight coughs. Use on the front of the chest, 3 times a day and at bedtime.

- Herbal inhalants; steams; body, hand, or footbaths; and massage oil made with aromatic essential oils such as eucalyptus, hyssop, thyme, peppermint, pine, rosemary, or yarrow flower are all excellent ways to support the immune system and bring comfort to the child.
- Use hydrotherapy by applying the wet sock treatment. After thoroughly warming the feet, put on cold, damp socks that have been moistened with yarrow flower tea. Put warm, dry wool socks over the damp socks, and put the child to bed. This will lessen congestion as the child sleeps.

BRUISES

Bruises are caused by blood that has escaped from broken vessels and has become trapped under the skin. They vary in size from very small to several inches and usually are black and blue; if they are close to the skin's surface they may be purplish. As they heal they often become yellowish green. Bruises usually are caused by trauma from bumps, falls, and bangs. If your child seems to bruise easily, consider nutritional deficiencies such as vitamin C, bioflavonoids, and vitamin K. If bruising appears spontaneously in areas that defy the likelihood of trauma, they may be a result of fragile capillaries caused by vitamin C or bioflavonoid deficiency, from blood vessels injured by infection or allergic reaction, or from a blood-clotting mechanism deficiency. Consult your physician.

Treatments

- See that the child's diet is high in bioflavonoid foods, such as red and yellow vegetables (squash, carrots, yams, beets),

leafy green vegetables (spinach, broccoli, chard), and fruits (blueberries, plums, cherries, grapes).
- Useful herbal medicines to offer as teas and herbal punches to strengthen the blood vessels include blueberry and huckleberry leaf, hawthorne berry or flowers, linden flowers, and meadowsweet.

Supplementation

Give immune-supporting vitamins and minerals in the following doses: vitamin C, 100 to 200 milligrams for children up to 18 months and 500 to 1,000 milligrams for older children; bioflavonoids, 50 to 100 milligrams for children up to 18 months and 100 to 500 milligrams for older children.

Homeopathy

Give arnica 6c immediately after trauma and then 3 times a day, for a few days.

Topical

- Apply cold compresses immediately after trauma for ½ hour. This will reduce the amount of bleeding and bruising.
- A warm application 24 hours after the trauma will increase the reabsorption of the bruise.
- Apply distilled witch hazel, arnica tincture, or St. John's wort oil to the area several times a day.
- Creams containing arnica, horse chestnut, or yarrow flower can be rubbed gently into the area.

Rub for Bruises
½ oz. witch hazel tincture
¼ oz. lobelia tincture

¼ oz. wormwood tincture

1 oz. water

Combine in a 2-ounce bottle; apply with a cotton ball, 3 times a day.

BURNS

Burns are injuries to the skin caused by excessive heat, chemicals, or electricity. The severity of a burn can vary. First-degree burns, such as a sunburn, are red or pink, swollen, and painful. Second-degree burns are red, swollen, painful, and blister immediately. Third-degree burns, which are the deepest, blacken, blister, or appear dead white. If an area receives a second-degree burn larger than the child's palm, or the child suffers from a third-degree burn of any size, consult your doctor. Remember to have the child drink lots of water whether treating at home or going to the doctor.

Treatments

- Immediately immerse the burned area in ice-cold water or use a wet ice compress for 15 to 30 minutes or until the pain has abated. Cover burn with loose dry gauze compresses. If compresses adhere to the burn, remove by moistening with comfrey/yarrow tea. Keep the burn clean and as sterile as possible to avoid infection.
- Apply fresh aloe gel from a plant or a prepared gel or juice. The plant will soothe the pain and burning and will act as an antiseptic to decrease risk of infection.
- Apply cool compresses made from an infusion of equal amounts of chamomile flowers, calendula flowers, yarrow flowers, peppermint, and comfrey leaf.

- Apply salves, oils, and creams a few hours after the burn occurs. Use calendula cream, vitamin E creams or oils, St. John's wort oil or salve, or comfrey salve or creams.
- Give a few drops of Bach Flower Rescue Remedy to the child and put a few drops into the cold-water soak.

CHICKEN POX

Chicken pox is a highly contagious viral infection of childhood. It spreads through droplets of saliva from coughing, sneezing, and talking. The child is most contagious just before the spots present until they have healed. Children between the ages of five and ten years old are at highest risk. The peak season for infection is late winter to spring. Incubation period after exposure is ten to twenty-one days, and most children are sick seven to ten days.

Chicken pox may start with a fever, cold, headache, or general malaise, but often a rash is the first sign. The rash begins on the trunk, face, scalp, ears, mucous membranes of the mouth, genitals and eyelids, and, rarely, the extremities. The rash consists of individual spots, which start out red and develop into fluid-filled vesicles that break and scab over. The blister-like spots are extremely itchy, and it is typical to have old and new spots at once. New spots continue to appear for the first three to four days of the illness. The fever can range from low to 104°F and is often worst on the third day of the rash.

It is best to discourage scratching of the spots, as this will result in scarring and increase the risk for secondary bacterial infection such as impetigo. Cutting the fingernails short and keeping them clean can be helpful.

On rare occasions, the complications of chicken pox can lead to encephalitis. If your child has a high fever, headache, vomiting, or extreme malaise, see a doctor. For spots that get infected or appear on the eyeball, consult a doctor.

The chicken pox virus is related to the virus that causes shingles in adults. It is not uncommon for a child with chicken pox to give an adult shingles.

Treatments

- Support the immune system with antiviral herbs such as echinacea, licorice, lemon balm, St. John's wort, and astragalus. Give immune-supporting foods, such as garlic, ginger, and Chinese mushrooms. Use immune-supporting vitamins and minerals, including vitamin C, beta-carotene, zinc, and bioflavonoids.
- For fever and general malaise use meadowsweet, chamomile, elder flowers, and linden flowers.
- Topically, use tepid herbal baths and washes made from burdock root, calendula flowers, chickweed, lavender flowers, nettles, or peppermint.
- To dry spots, use cotton balls to apply distilled witch hazel that has been refrigerated.
- Add 5 to 8 drops of essential oil of lavender, peppermint, or yarrow to 1 quart of tepid water. Apply with compresses or add to the bath.
- Creams made from comfrey, calendula, yarrow, and lavender can be used on the spots after the scabs have dried and fallen off. This will help heal the new skin and prevent scarring.
- If spots occur in the mouth or throat give a mouth rinse made from an infusion of goldenseal, witch hazel bark, and calendula flowers. Use ¼ cup of tea with ¼ cup of warm water and rinse several times a day. Swab the mouth lesions

with a mixture of equal amounts of tincture of peppermint and water. Use a cotton swab to apply to the sores several times a day.

COLD SORES

These small fluid-filled blisters ache, erupt, and crust over. They appear on the lips, nose, inside the mouth, or on the face. They are caused by the herpes simplex virus, which lives quietly on the nerve endings in the child's body after the initial infection. The initial attack is accompanied by fever, ulcers in the mouth or on the lips, swelling of the gums, and general malaise. When the immune resistance is lowered by stress, sun, fever, high sugar intake, fatigue, or immune stress, the quiet virus becomes active and causes a sore to appear.

Herpes simplex can spread so keep the child away from close contact with other children and small babies. Discourage scratching of the sores to avoid secondary bacterial infection. Keep the child out of bright sunlight to avoid worsening. If a sore appears on or near the eye, consult your doctor.

Treatments

- Internal treatments should be aimed at supporting the immune system, using herbs such as echinacea, astragalus, or usnea. To support the lymphatic system use herbs such as cleavers, burdock, calendula, or nettles. To decrease viral activity in the body use herbs such as licorice, lemon balm, St. John's wort, or venus flytrap.
- The following formula can be used as an infusion, taking 1 cup, 3 times a day, or as a tincture using ½ teaspoon, 3 times a day. Use during the infection and for 2 weeks

postinfection. Mix 1 part of each of the following: echinacea, lemon balm, and cleavers with ½ parts of licorice root, burdock, and calendula flowers.

- The amino acid lysine helps to inhibit the growth of the virus and can be used in supplement form at 250 milligrams, 3 times a day. Including in the child's diet foods that are high in lysine can be a great way to prevent reactivation of the virus. These include tuna, turkey, salmon, halibut, cheese, and yeast. Keep the diet low in foods that contain a high amount of the amino acid arginine, as it stimulates viral activity. The foods to avoid include nuts, seeds, chocolate, peanut butter, wheat, and beans.
- Optimal immune function depends on a diet high in fresh fruits, vegetables, whole grains, good proteins, and good fats and low in processed, preserved, refined foods; sugars; hydrogenated fats; and allergens. If your child has problems with cold sores make sure the diet is optimal.

Topical

- Apply a licorice and peppermint tea compress, or use equal parts of both tinctures and dab on cold sore with a cotton ball.
- Distilled witch hazel dabbed on several times a day in the blistering stage can ease the pain.
- Salves made from comfrey root, calendula flowers, St. John's wort, or vitamin E can be applied to the dry sores.

Herpes Lotion

Mix 3 drops each of the following essential oils: lavender, peppermint, and tea tree in 1 teaspoon of lemon balm tincture and 1 tablespoon of rosewater. Apply to blisters with a cotton ball several times a day.

COLIC

Colic is a cramp-like, intermittent abdominal pain that occurs mainly in babies and small children. Infantile colic or "three-month colic" seems to affect babies in the first weeks of life and may last three months. The baby seems to be in pain, possibly from the bowel, but it is really not clear what is the matter. Babies may cry inconsolably for hours a day, particularly in the evenings. They pull up their legs, clench their fists, and cry in discomfort. They may feed briefly but stop to return to crying. Rocking and cuddling will bring little comfort. In other respects, the child is normal. She gains weight well, has normal stools, and doesn't spit up regularly. Still, it is hard on the parents when the baby cannot be calmed.

A variation of the classical presentation of colic is the infant, more than two weeks old, who wakes every two hours, cries fretfully, takes a little formula or a minute at the breast, falls back into a fitful sleep, and wakes to repeat the sequence about two hours later.

Colic can be the symptom of emotional upset. A baby's close connection to his mother means he can sense if she is tense or worried. It is important to be calm and relaxed with the baby, not to be rushing around or uptight. If you are breast-feeding, make sure you are relaxed and not hurried when you are nursing.

Colic may be related to feeding problems. Breast-feeding mothers should check to see that the baby is latched on to the nipple properly. Be sure the baby is not making a loud sucking noise or gulping excessively. If bottle-feeding, check the bottle nipple to see if the hole is clogged, too big or too small, and that the latch is correct.

A baby's digestive system may be reacting to an irritant or allergen in the mother's breast milk or the formula, causing the colic to occur. Many babies react to cow's milk through the

Common Colic-Causing Foods

- Dairy
- Alcohol
- Coffee
- Chocolate
- Spicy foods and curries
- Garlic and onions
- Legumes and beans
- Too much fruit (especially grapes, peaches, plums, strawberries, pineapple)
- Cabbage family vegetables (broccoli, cabbage, cauliflower, brussels sprouts)

mother's breast milk, if the mother is eating dairy products, or in cow's milk–based formula. I recommend that breast-feeding moms avoid dairy products in their diet for at least three months. Other common food allergens that a baby may react to through breast milk include citrus fruits, wheat, and corn. Many foods may irritate the baby's digestion, even though she is not necessarily allergic to them. If you eliminate the most common colic-producing food and it persists, look to see what foods you eat most regularly or every day and eliminate those for a week to test.

Treatments

- Breast-feeding mothers can drink herbal teas made from catnip, cinnamon, dill, fennel, lemon balm, or crampbark. The medicinal properties will pass into the breast milk and on into the baby's stomach. Weak, diluted teas may be given directly to the baby by the dropperful every 15 minutes.

Seed Tea or Colic Water

Make an infusion from any one of the following essential oil–containing seeds: fennel, caraway seed, anise, or dill. Use 1 tablespoon of seeds to 8 ounces of water. Cover and steep for 10 minutes. Add 3 ounces of vegetable glycerine, and bottle. Use ¼ to ½ teaspoon every ½ hour if colicky or 15 minutes before feedings.

- Catnip used as an infusion acts as an antispasmodic and a carminative. It combines well with chamomile, crampbark, and fennel seed as a tea. It may also be used as tincture, 40 drops mixed with 1 ounce of water. Sweeten with rice syrup and give by the dropper every 15 minutes. A compress of warm catnip tea applied to the tummy can also bring comfort.

Lavender and Lobelia Fomentation

Make a strong infusion from lavender and lobelia. Soak a cloth in the warm infusion and apply over the tummy area with a hot water bottle or heating pad. If your baby has colicky episodes often, making an oil-based preparation can be an easy way to apply this treatment. Use lobelia infused in 2 ounces of olive oil and 20 drops of the essential oil of lavender.

- Herbal baths can reduce spasms and calm the baby. Relaxing herbs such as hops, lavender flowers, lemon balm, linden flowers, and skullcap can be made into infusions and added to a warm bath.

COMMON COLD

The common cold is a viral infection of the upper respiratory system. It usually involves discomfort of the throat, nose, sinuses, and sometimes the eyes (connected to the nose by the tear ducts), ears (connected to the nose by the eustachian tube), and lymph nodes of the neck (connected by the lymphatic channels). A cold is transmitted from person to person or from droplets on the hands or inanimate objects (toys, cups, handkerchiefs). The incubation period is two to seven days. A child is more likely to catch a cold when he is overtired, run-down, allergy-prone, or consumes a diet high in mucous-forming or immune-reducing foods, such as sugar, refined foods, and dairy products. Younger children and infants get more colds, as their immune systems are still maturing and not at full strength.

Cold symptoms include nasal congestion; sneezing; clear nasal discharge; a sore, scratchy throat; and a fever up to 103°F. Other minor symptoms include watery red eyes, coughing, ear pain, and enlarged lymph glands in the neck. Colds can lead to other respiratory illnesses such as bronchitis, ear infections, laryngitis, sinusitis, and pharyngitis.

Treatments

- Give immune-supporting vitamins and minerals in the following doses: vitamin C, 200 to 500 milligrams, 3 times a day; zinc, 10 to 15 milligrams, daily; bioflavonoids, 100 to 500 milligrams, daily.
- Give lots of fluids. Have the child sip water, diluted fruit juice, or herbal teas or punches frequently. This keeps the throat moist, the body hydrated, and checks the fever. Use herbal teas of aniseed, chamomile, catnip, elder flowers, eyebright, hyssop, lemon balm, licorice root, meadowsweet,

mints, nettles, red clover flowers, thyme, and yarrow flowers. Herbal popsicles made from medicinal herbs and fruit
juice are a great way to offer fluids and cool the discomfort
in the throat and mouth. Use teas made from cleavers, elder
flowers, spearmint, licorice, lemon balm, wintergreen, red
clover, ginger, and linden flowers.

- Support the immune system with immune-enhancing herbs
  and help to resolve the infection with antiviral herbs such
  as licorice, lemon balm, echinacea, usnea, astragalus, and
  garlic. With a fever, combine with linden flowers, yarrow
  flowers, catnip, meadowsweet, or elder flowers.

Elixir for Colds
1 part echinacea tincture
1 part garlic syrup
1 part thyme tincture
1 part licorice tincture
1 part lemon balm tincture or glycerite
1 part linden flower tincture
½ part ginger syrup
½ part elder flowers tincture

Give ½ to 1 teaspoon, 4 times a day. This same formula
can be made as an infusion and sweetened with honey.

- Herbal baths may be used to decongest, relax, warm, and
  reduce aches and pains. Use infusions of the aromatic herbs
  like eucalyptus, lavender, marjoram, peppermint, or thyme.
  Combine with relaxing herbs like chamomile, hops, and linden flowers.
- Chest rubs increase circulation and warm and relax the
  chest and respiratory muscles. They are best applied topically before bed or napping, then cover the chest with a cotton T-shirt. Rubs usually contain aromatic herbs such as

eucalyptus, hyssop, thyme, peppermint, camphor, or rose-mary, which are very volatile and therefore penetrate the skin easily, stimulate blood flow, relax the muscles, and deliver medication to the local area. They can be especially effective with spastic, tight coughs.

- Herbal steams also deliver the medication to the local area. Again, aromatic volatile herbs are used, as they are very antiseptic and help to disinfect the respiratory passages. A favorite steam of mine is the combination of 1 teaspoon each of chamomile flowers, yarrow flowers, and lavender flowers.
- Humidify the child's room and put hyssop, peppermint, eucalyptus, or yarrow oil in the humidifier as an antispasmodic.

CONJUNCTIVITIS

Conjunctivitis, or pinkeye, is a bacterial or viral infection of the conjunctiva, the transparent membrane that covers the white of the eye and lines the eyelid. Conjunctivitis causes redness of the entire white of the eye and the accumulation of a yellow pus-like discharge, often gluing the eye shut after sleep. The eyelids may swell and redden, and there is a burning or gritty sensation in the eye. Vision is normal, and light usually does not bother the eye.

Conjunctivitis is highly contagious, spreading by contact with discharge from the eye or via objects (washcloths, handkerchiefs, or toys) that have been handled by the contagious child. Conjunctivitis in one eye spreads quickly to the other eye.

Conjunctivitis may exist alone or can accompany a sore throat, cold, tonsillitis, or sinusitis. If conjunctivitis is chronic, consider food allergy or airborne allergy to chemicals, dusts, or pollens.

Treatments

- Have your child wash his hands frequently, avoid touching or rubbing the eyes, and wash away any discharge with warm water and cotton balls. Always wipe from the nose side of the eye to the outside, using a clean cotton ball for each wipe. Always treat both eyes even if only one is pink. If you are breast-feeding put a few drops of breast milk into the eyes.
- Give immune-supporting herbs and supplements orally to help the body fight the infection and to prevent spreading of the infection. (See Part II, Working with the Young Immune System, starting on page 19.)
- Herbal eyewashes made from infusions can be used as a wash in an eyecup or a few drops can be put into the eye. Eyebright is useful in reducing inflammation and irritation of the eye. It can be combined with raspberry leaf. Raspberry's astringent action helps to fight the local infection and decrease redness of the eye. Combine both of these with goldenseal for its antimicrobial action and its tonifying effect on the mucous membranes of the eyes. This combination is very helpful most of the time.

CONSTIPATION

Most children have a bowel movement every day or so and sometimes more. Breast-fed babies may not have a stool every day, yet they are not necessarily constipated. However, if the stool is hard and delayed in passing, then constipation is present. Commonly, constipation is combined with other digestive disturbances such as stomachache, cramps, loss of appetite, and sometimes vomiting in babies.

Constipation can be due to an organic physical cause or a functional cause. Organic causes are rare and relatively easy to diagnose. Most cases of constipation are functional and involve no physical abnormality. The function of the large colon is to store unabsorbed food waste and to absorb and conserve water from the liquid material received from the small intestines. Factors that favor the absorption of too much water by the colon lead to constipation. Determining what the underlying factors are is important to the resolution of the constipation.

Dietary factors that play a role in constipation include a diet low in roughage or whole fibers. Fibers play a role in keeping the stool moist and soft as well as acting as a bulking agent that helps to stimulate peristaltic movement of the colon. Food allergies may present as constipation and should be ruled out. (See Food Allergy, page 31.) Animal products, such as meat, cheese, and milk, can lead to colon irritation and reduced peristaltic movement. A diet high in white flour, sugars, and processed foods gives little roughage and works against good colon health.

Irregular bowel habits can also be a factor. It is important to encourage the child not to resist or ignore the normal impulse to have a bowel movement. If the child is preoccupied with other tasks or feels rushed, he or she is more likely to resist the urge. If the child has experienced passing a painful, hard stool, he or she is often even more reluctant to have bowel movements. Sometimes toilet training can be emotionally upsetting to the child, which may lead to avoidance of passing stool. Worry, tension, and anxiety may all lead to reduced bowel movements. Many children feel stress in their digestive tract, leading to bowel tension and spastic pain of the colon. Often, times of change or transition (starting school, moving to a new home, changing schools) will bring on episodes of constipation.

Low amounts of water and other fluids in the diet can lead to dry, hard stools. If your child is prone to constipation, encourage him to drink lots of fluids, including water, herbal teas, and fruit juices throughout the day.

Lack of exercise can contribute to constipation. Exercise promotes blood circulation to the colon, allowing the bowel muscles to be nourished and oxygenated so they can function properly. Encourage your child to be active and not overly sedentary.

Constipation sometimes accompanies other types of illness such as fever, headache, and vomiting. The child's bowel habits may otherwise be normal. In this case, use mild bowel-stimulating herbs to encourage returning to the normal pattern after resolution of the illness.

Sometimes, constipation is associated with deficiencies of nutrients like vitamin C and magnesium. Increase foods rich in these nutrients in the child's diet and consider supplementation. (See Part III, Nutrition for Infants and Children, starting on page 37.)

Constipation overdistends the large bowel, causing a loss of muscle tone, and the impulse to empty the bowel becomes even weaker. This cycle can lead to chronic constipation. The sooner you can help your child resolve the constipation and establish regular bowel movements, the better. Chronic constipation will result in altering the gut flora and lead to breakdown of the gut wall, which may lead to allergic problems, skin rash, headaches, and chronic digestive complaints.

Treatments

- Make sure the diet is high in fresh fruits, vegetables (raw and cooked), and whole grains and cereals. These foods provide good-quality fibers that help to bulk the stool and stimulate peristalsis in the colon. Include foods such as nuts, seeds, figs, prunes, raisins, apricots, applesauce, rhubarb, blackberries, oat bran, and whole-grain cereals.
- Make bowel habits regular and get the child in the habit of responding to the urge for stool. If the child is young, it

may be helpful to have him or her sit on the toilet regularly at the same time each day; after meals is a good time to do this. This will encourage the occurrence of a regular urge. Make sure the child is not rushed or hurried and there is enough time to sit five to ten minutes each day.

- Encourage regular activity—playing outside, playing sports, running, swimming, and bike riding.
- Improve the bowel microflora with acidophilus supplementation, 1 or 2 capsules before bed, yogurt with live cultures, and other probiotic foods.
- Massage the abdomen with warm castor oil with a few drops of the essential oil of rosemary, lavender, or marjoram. Lobelia oil can also be used. Remember when massaging the abdomen to work in a clockwise fashion so as to stay with the normal direction of the colon.

Herbal Laxatives

The use of strong herbal laxatives is usually not needed. In any case, they should only be used infrequently. The herbal approach should be to try to soften the stool, restore peristalsis, and relax tension from the colon. This can be done by combining several herbs into a remedy. The following herbal groups should be represented in the remedy.

Herbal bulk laxatives are herbs that soften, moisten, and bulk out the colon to support peristalsis and move the stool along. Add psyllium seed or flaxseed to hot cereals, or soak a teaspoon of seeds in a cup of hot water and sip each morning.

Herbal bowel stimulants can be used to increase liver function, stimulate the bowel wall, and encourage passing of the stool. Many mild herbal bowel stimulants can be used safely with children. They should be employed with other bowel-supporting measures such as diet, water intake, and exercise. Many of these plants stimulate bile secretions from the liver, a normal inducement for the bowels to move. Choose herbs such as dandelion root, fennel seed, licorice root, or yellow dock. Use them as decoctions sweetened with honey, or use 10 to 20 drops of tincture in warm water, 3 times a day.

Herbal bowel relaxants are very useful in reducing tension and spasm in the colon. They relax the bowel tissue and calm the child's tension or uneasiness about having a bowel movement. Use herbs like chamomile, catnip, crampbark, hops, lemon balm, and lobelia regularly in herbal teas or punches, or give them as tinctures and glycerites.

If using lobelia for severe cramping or colon tension, mix 1 teaspoon of tincture with 1 teaspoon of ginger tincture; put in a 1-ounce amber bottle, and fill with distilled water. Administer 5 to 10 drops, as needed.

Herbal Bowel Relaxant
1 part catnip
1 part crampbark
1 part fennel seed
½ part hops

Prepare as a tea, tincture, or glycerite. (See Making Herbal Preparations, page 259.)

Herbal mucilages found in herbs such as marshmallow root, slippery elm, or Irish moss bring water into the colon and soften the stool. They also lubricate and decrease irritation of the colon wall. A gruel made from 1 teaspoon of slippery elm powder mixed with 1 tablespoon of warm water and a pinch of cinnamon can be eaten daily to moisten the stool and encourage bowel movements. (See Syrup of Marshmallow recipe, page 266.)

COUGH

Coughing is a natural reflex that guards the respiratory tract from foreign materials that may block or irritate the air passages. Most often, coughing is beneficial as a way to clear the respiratory passages. However, there are times when coughing is ineffective. It interferes with sleep, causes exhaustion from muscular effort, and may even lead to vomiting. Coughs may be dry and irritating or loose and productive. In the latter instance, the coughing causes the movement of mucus that has been loosened by the secretions. A dry, irritating cough can be due to infection or inflammation in the nose, sinus, ear, or throat; a foreign body; chemicals; secondary smoke or environmental irritations; or nervousness and tension. A loose, wet cough can be caused by bronchial infection or inflammation, or bronchial constriction or allergy. It is important to choose a remedy to fit the type and cause of the cough. A cough that worsens at night when in bed is more often due to infection, irritation, or inflammation in the upper respiratory tract, which causes fluids to trigger the reflex when lying down. A cough in the lower respiratory tract is generally present at all times of the day and night.

It is important to find the underlying cause of the cough and treat that. Causes can include allergy, infection, poor bowel function, stress, emotional need, nutritional deficiencies, poor diet, asthma, secondary smoke exposure, or inhaled foreign objects.

Treatments

The goal of the treatment should be to assist the body in its own healing process; to aid the respiratory passages in clearing the infection, inflammation, or irritation; to soothe and heal the respiratory mucous membranes; and to support the immune system in bringing wellness back to the body. A cough remedy can loosen a tight, dry cough; dry up a wet, congested cough;

decrease coughing spasms; and reduce the frequency of a cough. It is generally not a good idea to suppress a cough, as it is a defensive mechanism for the body. Yet, at times it can be beneficial to reduce the frequency of a cough at night to aid in sleeping and to ensure a restful night for child and parents.

- Herbs that loosen and expel mucus from the chest are classified as expectorants. These plants increase watery secretions, loosening and stimulating the movement of catarrh from the lungs. In other words, they make the cough reflex more productive. Expectorant herbs include hyssop, elecampane, thyme, aniseed, and mullein.
- Herbs that are helpful in relieving a dry, irritated cough, by soothing the irritated mucous membranes and increasing the excretion of mucus, include licorice, marshmallow root, plantain, slippery elm, and elecampane. If irritations are due to a nervous tickle in the throat, include one of the following in your formula: crampbark, lemon balm, skullcap, or linden flowers.

Cough Syrup for Dry Cough (available from Gaia's Children) is a great premixed formula that is available in many health food stores and co-ops. It is a base of loquat syrup with the following herbal extracts mixed in: plantain leaf, mullein leaf and flower, Irish moss, marshmallow root, aniseed, pleurisy root, crampbark, and gingerroot.

Cough Syrup for Wet Cough (available from Gaia's Children) is formulated for a cough that is wet, or, in other words, there is mucus in the lungs and the child sounds phlegmy. Use as directed on the label. It also is in a loquat base with the following herbal extracts mixed in: elecampane root, licorice root, aniseed, thyme leaf, crampbark, wild cherry bark, cinnamon bark, and hyssop herb.

Nutrition

Avoiding foods that increase mucous production or inhibit immune response is an important part of treating cough. These include dairy products, refined carbohydrates, refined sugars, excessive fruit juices, and hydrogenated fats. Include foods that support the immune system, increase circulation to the chest, and supply necessary vitamins and minerals, such as garlic, onion, vegetable broths, ginger, and lots of fluids.

Helpful immune-supporting supplements include zinc, beta-carotene, vitamin C, bioflavonoids, and essential fatty acids.

Herbal Remedies

Tea for Dry Cough

Use 1 teaspoon each of licorice root, marshmallow root, aniseed, and cinnamon bark. Add to 16 ounces of cold water, simmer gently covered for 10 minutes. Strain and sweeten, if desired.

Tea for Loose, Wet Cough

Use 1 teaspoon each of mullein, thyme, aniseed, and plantain leaves. Pour 16 ounces of boiling water over the herbs and cover. Steep for 5 minutes, strain, and sweeten, if desired.

For infants, dilute tea with an equal amount of water and give in a bottle, cup, or by teaspoon doses every 2 hours. For children use 1 cup, 3 times a day.

Herbal cough syrups can be simple to make and easy to administer due to their pleasant taste. Onion or garlic syrup (see recipes on pages 265 and 219, respectively) can be effective in treating upper and lower respiratory coughs. Either of the previously described tea recipes can be made into a syrup by taking the strained tea, adding an equal amount of raw sugar, and boiling hard for 5 minutes. Cool and bottle. Store in the refrigerator.

For infants use 10 to 30 drops in a little water, 3 or 4 times a day. For children use ½ to 1 teaspoon, 3 or 4 times a day.

Chest rubs are useful in increasing circulation and in warming and relaxing the chest and respiratory muscles. They are best applied topically before bed or napping. Then cover the chest with a cotton T-shirt. Rubs usually contain aromatic herbs such as eucalyptus, hyssop, thyme, peppermint, camphor, or rosemary, which are very volatile and therefore penetrate the skin easily, stimulate blood flow, relax the muscles, and deliver medication to the local area. They can be especially effective with spastic, tight coughs.

Herbal steams can be used to deliver medication to the local area. Again, the aromatic, volatile herbs are used (see previous section), as they are all very antiseptic and help to disinfect the respiratory passages. A favorite steam is a combination of a teaspoon each of chamomile flowers, yarrow flowers, and lavender flowers.

CRADLE CAP

Cradle cap is marked by a thick, waxy, yellowish encrustation that appears on the baby's scalp, particularly on the top of the head. Cradle cap is caused by the hyperactivity of the glands in the scalp that secrete sebum. It can appear in the first few months of life and last until two or three years of age. It is a seborrhic condition of the skin and can be accompanied by seborrhic dermatitis, which is an eczema that affects the eyebrows, forehead, and behind the ears. This has been associated with low levels of zinc, magnesium, and biotin. It can also be associated with intolerance to formula or a food eaten by the breast-feeding mother.

Treatments

- If the case is mild, one of the following remedies should be helpful. If the cradle cap is moderate to severe, I would also recommend trying a hypoallergenic formula, such as Alimentum or Nutramogen, or, if breast-feeding, reviewing your diet for possible food sensitivity. Supplementation of zinc, magnesium, biotin, and essential fatty acids to baby or mother can be helpful. Brushing regularly with a soft baby brush will help to remove the crust.
- Astringent decoctions made from herbs such as witch hazel bark, white oak bark, and burdock root are used as washes to slow down glandular production. They can be used as a rinse to follow shampooing. They are left on the scalp and not rinsed out.

Cradle Cap Scalp Rinse
Infusion of 2 parts red clover
2 parts viola tricolor leaves
1 part burdock seeds

Let the herbs steep for 10 to 15 minutes before straining. Use to rinse the scalp several times a week. Leave on scalp. Do not rinse out.

Scalp Oil 1
An oil rub of 2 ounces of olive oil and 5 drops of lavender, rosemary, or basil essential oils may be used. Apply to

baby's head before going to bed. In the morning, wash off with a mild calendula shampoo on a washcloth. Rub gently and remove the crust.

Scalp Oil 2

Make an herbal oil as described in Part VI, page 262, of nettles, chamomile, and burdock seed. Warm the oil slightly and apply at night to the baby's scalp. Remove in the morning as described in the previous section.

CROUP

Croup is a common childhood illness that is contracted in the same manner as a cold: by airborne droplets or by direct contact with an infected person. It is an infection of the vocal cords and surrounding areas, causing swelling and inflammation. Croup is usually viral in origin and most often occurs in children three months to three years of age. As with many viral infections, croup occurs most often in the fall and winter. This is usually not a life-threatening disease, but it is nonetheless one of the most frightening of the childhood diseases.

Croup is characterized by a tight, dry, brassy, barking cough. The child develops difficulty breathing, with more pronounced difficulty when inhaling rather than exhaling, often with a distinct crowing sound on inhalation. These symptoms are caused from the swelling and inflammation in the vocal cord region. Fever is usually absent or low grade (101°F), and congestion due to increased mucous production can cause airway obstruction.

Typically, a child with croup will awaken in the night. Episodes can last several hours, subside, and return again the next night. The symptoms of croup can be mild or severe and can reoccur with each upper respiratory infection the child catches. Croup might also be a one-time occurrence.

Choking on an aspirated foreign object may present with a croup-like cough but can be ruled out because a croupy child can talk between episodes of coughing, while a choking child is unable to talk at all. Acute epiglottis, a severe, rapidly progressive bacterial infection, can be life-threatening due to airway obstruction. The epiglottis, located at the base of the tongue, becomes swollen and red, accompanied by a sudden high fever (103°F to 105°F) with difficulty breathing and swallowing. This is a medical emergency and immediate medical treatment is needed. Call your doctor or visit the emergency room if you suspect this illness.

Treatments

- Stay calm, do not panic, and try to calm and console your child. Getting upset will only make matters worse.
- Sit the child up, give sips of Composition Essence for Children (available from Gaia's Children; see Herbal First-Aid Remedies, page 16) diluted in warm water, and rub the chest, back, neck, and throat with an aromatic chest rub. (See page 112.)
- Warm steam from a humidifier will help, or run a hot shower and sit in a closed bathroom quietly, with the child breathing slowly and deeply. Add a few drops of a warming, relaxing, herbal essential oil to the steam to help ease breathing. Try a few drops of rosemary, lavender, or thyme oil.
- Cool moist air can also be helpful. Try opening a window or wrapping the child up warmly and taking him or her outside to sit for a while. The coolness reduces swelling and

inflammation. Cool-mist humidifiers can also used in the child's bedroom.

- Give several drops of Bach Flower Rescue Remedy directly into the mouth or in a small amount of water to help ease the child's fear and anxiety. A dose may be given every hour during a croupy episode if needed.
- Give sips of warm herbal infusions made from soothing demucent, antispasmodic, and anti-inflammatory herbs, such as licorice root, marshmallow root, catnip, crampbark, thyme, and wild cherry bark.
- Mix equal parts of tincture of catnip, skullcap, licorice root, hyssop, and peppermint. Add 3 to 20 drops, depending on age, to 2 ounces of warm water. Give 1 tablespoon every 15 minutes until the breathing gets easier.
- The following day, give the child lots of fluids, warm herbal teas, lemon and honey, or warm diluted fruit juice. Have him or her eat lightly, avoiding dairy products, sugars, and fats.
- Before bed, give the child a warm bath with aromatic oils like lavender or eucalyptus. Rub her throat and chest with a warming, vaporous chest rub. Keep the air in the bedroom moist and fresh by cracking a window and using a humidifier. This may prevent another episode during the night.

Aromatic Chest Rub

Add 5 drops of the following essential oils: oil of pine, lavender flowers, thyme, peppermint, and yarrow flowers to 2 ounces of melted cocoa butter after it has been removed from the heat. Mix well while still warm and put into a 2-ounce container to cool. (Gaia's Children makes a Warming Vaporous Chest rub with the same essential oils but a more complex base, which can be purchased at your local health food store.)

CUTS

A minor cut or graze can be treated at home if it has not affected the muscles, tendons, or bones and there is no risk of tetanus. If the cut is deep and gaping, see your doctor; stitching may be necessary. Natural remedies, however, may still be used to reduce pain and assist in healing.

Treatments

- Clean the area well with calendula or tea tree soap and warm water. Apply an herbal antiseptic wash made from calendula flowers, echinacea, goldenseal, myrrh, yarrow flowers, or tea tree oil. Either use a tea or 5 to 10 drops of tincture in warm water.
- Apply a cream or salve made from comfrey, calendula, St. John's wort, or yarrow and cover with a bandage. Use the antiseptic wash once a day to prevent infection.
- Give Bach Flower Rescue Remedy for the trauma of the fall or bang. Arnica 6c or 12c will be helpful in reducing swelling and increasing healing.

DIAPER RASH

Rashes in the diaper area may occur for several reasons: infrequently changed wet diapers, detergent, fabric, bleach, chemicals, yeast infection, bacterial infection, ammonia in urine, food allergy, eczema, or plastic sensitivity. Diaper rashes are red, chafed, irritated skin in the diaper area. A herpes infection or impetigo can come secondarily to the diaper rash.

Regular, frequent changing of diapers and good bottom care are essential for managing diaper rash. Wash your baby's bottom with herbal teas made from calendula flowers, comfrey leaf, chamomile flowers, and lavender flowers or with herbal waters such as rose or lavender. The bottom should be dried well and left to air dry a few minutes before diapering. Applying an herbal cream or oil lightly over the bottom will protect it from urine and stool, soothe the irritation, and heal the skin. If using herbal body powders remember to dust the bottom lightly 1 or 2 times a day, but avoid caking or overuse. One-way diaper liners aid in keeping the bottom dry.

Treatments

- Wash the skin at each changing with herbal infusions made from any of these herbs: calendula flowers, chamomile flowers, witch hazel, rosemary, yarrow flowers, or comfrey leaf. Creams or salves made of comfrey, St. John's wort, chickweed, or plantain should be applied after washing and drying with each diaper changing.
- Use herbal oils made from herbs like St. John's wort, plantain, or comfrey instead of creams or salves.
- If yeast is the cause, add 5 to 10 drops of thyme, oregano, or sage essential oil to 1 ounce of calendula cream. If bacterial infection is the cause, use a goldenseal and myrrh wash, followed by a cream with 5 to 10 drops of lavender or rosemary essential oil.

DIARRHEA

Diarrhea refers to the consistency of the stool and not the frequency of the bowel movements. The number of bowel movements each day measures the severity of the diarrhea. Diarrhea occurs commonly in children during an acute illness and usually resolves in twenty-four hours.

Diarrhea in the infant often has mucus mixed with it and is watery and runny. It may be accompanied by cramps, loss of appetite, vomiting, and fever. Prolonged diarrhea in an infant can lead to dehydration, weight loss, and poor growth patterns. The usual causes of diarrhea are infections of the digestive tract and intolerance to foods. In infants, infections may be caused by respiratory viruses as well as intestinal viruses, bacteria, and parasites. Large amounts of foods such as fruits may trigger diarrhea in some babies. Foods that the baby may not tolerate or be allergic to will often trigger diarrhea. Antibiotic treatments used for babies often cause diarrhea as a side effect.

Diarrhea in children over the age of five differs in several respects from that which occurs in babies. The likelihood of dehydration decreases with the increasing age and size of the child. Serious dehydration is unlikely after age five, unless diarrhea is prolonged and accompanied by vomiting. Intestinal viruses are the most common cause of diarrhea in older children, followed by bacterial infection, candida infection, or intestinal parasites. Older children are less likely to get diarrhea from respiratory viruses and food intolerances. Don't assume that a food intolerance has resolved if diarrhea goes away. More likely, there is a new, deeper symptom such as inflammatory intestinal disease, producing symptoms of gas, bloating, and vague abdominal discomfort.

Overeating of allergenic foods or fats that are hard to digest and can irritate the digestive tract can cause diarrhea and emptying of the colon. Foods rich in butter, fried foods, creamy sauces, whipped cream, spices, excessive fruits, fruit juices, milk, or ice cream can produce this effect. Emotional upset, stress, anxiety, and overexcitement can all cause diarrhea with stomachache. This can be an isolated episode or a more frequent pattern, reflecting a stressful issue for your child, perhaps school. Treatment here should include the use of herbs like chamomile, lemon balm, linden flowers, oats, skullcap, and valerian.

Food poisoning will cause frequent diarrhea every half hour or so, often accompanied by stomach pains, nausea, vomiting, fever, and malaise. Precooked foods and undercooked meats and eggs are common carriers of salmonella. Listeria infection can be gotten through some types of cheese.

Chronic diarrhea is usually more mild and appears periodically between times of normally formed stool. This is a sign that the digestive tract is not functioning properly and has irritated mucous membranes. Food allergy or intolerance is often the cause. This creates constant irritation to the digestive lining and starts to disrupt the normal bowel microflora and digestive secretions, leading to abnormal digestive patterns. To treat this type of diarrhea, eliminate food intolerances, restore digestive microflora with acidophilus supplementation, restore digestive enzymes, and heal the mucous membranes of the intestines with appropriate herbs.

Treatments

Avoid all foods and give only fluids except for milk, which will aggravate the diarrhea. Use fruit juices made from blackberry, apple, pear, or raspberry for their astringent properties. Warm the juices and herbal teas, as cold drinks will aggravate the digestive tract. If no fever is present and the child asks for food, give brown rice gruel, plain yogurt with live cultures, or warm broths.

For Infants Under Three Months Old

- Continue nursing.
- Give Pedialite for 24 hours. Use as directed on the bottle.

- Oil the skin over the abdomen with olive oil and essential oil of lavender.
- Give anise, chamomile, or meadowsweet as infusions, ½ teaspoon every 30 to 60 minutes.
- Nursing mothers should take herbal astringent teas and tinctures such as raspberry leaf, meadowsweet, or rosemary.

For Infants Three to Twelve Months Old

- Continue nursing.
- Give clear liquids, vegetable broths, or herbal teas.
- Avoid milk products.
- Give acidophilus supplementation.
- Apply castor oil packs to the abdomen.

For Children One to Three Years Old

- Give clear liquids.
- Give vegetable broths or herbal teas.
- Avoid milk products.
- Give acidophilus supplementation.
- Apply castor oil packs to the abdomen.
- Give herbal astringent tinctures—blackberry, rosemary, or meadowsweet.
- Give clay water (1 teaspoon bentonite to 6 ounces water, 1 to 3 times per day).

For Children Three Years and Older

- Slippery elm powder may be given as a gruel or tea. Mixing it with an equal part of carob powder may also be helpful. Give small amounts every few hours.

- Give an infusion of one of the berry leaves, such as strawberry, blackberry, or raspberry. These are high in tannins and have an astringent effect on the digestive tract. Use 1 teaspoon of leaves per cup and give in 1 tablespoon doses, every 1 to 2 hours.
- Unsweetened carob powder may either be mixed with a bit of water or blackberry root tea to make a paste, or it can be added to applesauce. Use ½ to 1 teaspoon per dose, every 2 hours.
- Make a decoction of blackberry root or blackberry root syrup. Use ¼ to ½ cup of the decoction or ½ to 1 teaspoon of the syrup, 3 to 4 times a day.
- Offer rosemary tea, ¼ to ½ cup, twice a day, or 2 tablespoons, every 2 hours.
- Administer ginger drops. Mix 1 teaspoon of ginger tincture with 2 tablespoons of filtered water in a 1-ounce bottle. Give doses of 3 to 5 drops, every 1 to 2 hours.
- Give rice water. Cook 1 cup of rice in 4 cups of water; strain the liquid off; and give ½ cup, 3 times a day.
- Marshmallow decoction or syrup can be given if there is a lot of burning when passing stool. The marshmallow will soothe the irritated tissue and will also absorb some of the excess water in the colon.

EAR INFECTION

Earache is one of the most common reasons children see the doctor. Ear pain may be caused by infection or by fluid and swelling in the ears, sinuses, or throat. If it occurs in the outer ear canal it is called *otitis extrena*. Infection may be caused by a foreign object, boil, eczema, or excessive scratching of the canal. Earaches occur at any age but tend to be more frequent up to the age of eight years old. This is partly because the head is not fully grown and the eustachian tube has a poor angle for drainage. In small children and infants, earaches and infections might be missed or silent, as the child is less able to communicate what the problem is. Crying and pulling at the ear may be the only clues.

Middle ear infection, called *otitis media*, occurs in the part of the ear directly behind the eardrum. It is due to an inflammatory state of the tissue lining the eustachian tube, middle ear, and throat. This leads to eustachian tube blockage, causing a decrease in the drainage of the fluid, which in turn leads to a buildup of fluids, causing an increase in pressure, growth of bacteria, and possible rupture of the eardrum. A middle ear infection often accompanies colds, upper respiratory infections, sinusitis, and throat infections. It may also be associated with infants who are put to bed with a bottle as they fall asleep. Common symptoms associated with an ear infection include crying and pulling at the ear, ear pain, pain in the throat with swallowing, drainage of pus or bloody discharge from the ear, fever, and swollen tonsils and glands. Often, the fever drops during the day and rises back up in the evening. Ear pressure is increased when lying down, which is why the child wakes from sleep crying in pain. Prop the child or the bed up to bring the head higher than the torso.

Serous otitis media, or fluid in the ear without infection, will cause intermittent pain as the pressure behind the eardrum rises and falls with position and activity. The fluid often gets thick and diminishes hearing in that ear. This condition leads to frequent episodes of acute middle ear infection and is associated with allergies, food intolerances, and chronically swollen tonsils and adenoids. The standard treatment is to put little tubes through the eardrum to allow drainage of the fluid. The use of tubes can be avoided with treatment of the root cause of the membrane swelling.

Common causes associated with chronic swelling of the mucous membranes and fluid in the ear include any of the following.

- Teething
- Allergies to foods such as milk, cheese, ice cream, citrus, eggs, peanuts; secondary smoke from tobacco or wood-stoves; airbornes such as pollens, dust, animal danders, or molds; or chemicals and food additives and colorings might cause fluid in the ear. The allergic response leads to a narrowing or collapse of the eustachian tube and swelling of the tonsils and adenoids, leading to impaired lymphatic drainage, obstruction, and more fluid in the ear.
- Common nutritional deficiencies associated with chronic fluid in the ear include zinc and omega 3 and 6 oils. They play an important role in immune function and the health of the mucous membranes.
- Mechanical obstruction may be caused by biomechanical problems with structural components surrounding the ears, neck, and head. This can lead to nervous impairment and inhibition of the local immune response. If your child has had head trauma, a forceps or vacuum-assisted delivery, or a hard, long pushing stage of birth and has earaches that do not respond to treatments, consider having him or her visit a cranial sacral therapist. This type of manipulation of the head can help to correct any mechanical problems.

Finding the cause of the fluid will help you to choose the best treatment. Addressing food intolerances is particularly important. The younger the child, the younger the digestive tract, and the more likely it is that it will not tolerate a specific food. Children with an allergic family history are likely to experience food intolerance. When treating chronic fluid in the middle ear, I always eliminate any food that is at high risk for being an aller-

See your doctor if the following conditions are present:

- Ear pain lasts longer than one hour.
- Temperature is higher than 103°F.
- Ear discharge is present.

gen even if the child is not truly allergic. These foods become added stresses to the immune system and digestive tract, making them harder to heal.

Antibiotics are frequently used to treat ear infections and many parents find their child on repeated courses. Antibiotics will work if there is an infection of the ear, but if there is pain, fluid, and increased pressure, they will not be effective, as they are not decongestants or anti-inflammatories. The mistreatment of *serous otitis media* with antibiotics can lead to weakening of the immune system and recurring infection. Once a child has been treated with antibiotics for an ear infection, she is more likely to need them again in a few months.

Unless the infection is severe with a high fever and does not respond to a day or two of herbal treatment, many middle ear infections can be managed without the use of antibiotics. Naturopathic doctors can often help to resolve an acute middle ear infection safely without them.

Treatments

If the child has recurring infections, chronic fluid in the ear, or an allergic family history, use good dietary habits as described in the chapter on nutrition. Put the child on extra immune nutrients such as beta-carotene, zinc, vitamin C, omega 3 and 6 essential

Hints for Soothing Ear Pain

- Place the child in an upright position.
- Use heat on the ear and neck. A hot water bottle, warm compress, or heating pad can be used. Apply the heat for 10 to 20 minutes, several times a day.
- A baked or blanched onion poultice can be very soothing and helps to break up congestion with its warm sulfur vapors. Take a medium-size onion and bake in the oven for 15 minutes or blanch in boiling water for a minute. Wrap it in gauze and place over the ear or behind it.
- Add a few drops of lavender and rosemary essential oils to warm olive oil and apply around the ears, throat, and nose.
- Administer warm ear drops. Ear drops made from herbal oils or glycerites can be helpful in reducing the infection, fluid, or both. Glycerine absorbs water, so I often choose glycerine drops for treating chronic fluid problems. Always warm the drops to body temperature before applying, as cold in the ear will increase the pain. Never use any ear drops if the eardrum is ruptured or you see discharge coming from the ear.

fatty acids, and bioflavonoids. Use herbs that build up the immune system (astragalus, chamomile, garlic, ginger, hyssop, licorice, reishi mushrooms, usnea), heal the mucous membranes (elder flowers, eyebright, ribwort), and increase lymphatic drainage (calendula, cleavers, nettles). Use these treatments for several months and through the cold season. If the child gets an acute infection use some of the suggestions in the following section to resolve the episode.

Basic Ear Oil
Use equal parts mullein oil, St. John's wort oil, and calendula succus. Add garlic oil for acute bacterial infection or to prevent the onset of infection. Goldenseal glycerite is also good for acute bacterial infection and to tonify the membranes. A few drops of ephedra tincture or lobelia oil may be used for narrowing of the eustachian tube, as this will relax and open the tube. Lobelia will also reduce severe pain. Ribwort and goldenseal glycerite drops can also be used for chronic catarrh and fluid in the ear.

Treat the acute infection with frequent doses of immune-supporting herbs such as echinacea, astragalus, garlic, chamomile, or wild indigo. Give a dose every 2 hours while the infection is acute. When the child starts to recover, administer a dose 3 times a day. Also include lymphatic- and mucous membrane–supporting herbs such as calendula flowers, cleavers, eyebright, elder flowers, and ribwort.

Liquid echinacea and vitamin C, a product by Naturopathic Formulas, available in many health food stores, combines echinacea and ginger with immune supplements such as vitamin C, bioflavonoids, zinc, beta-carotene, and vitamin B6. This excellent product will boost the immune response to infection.

See treatment for fever, sore throat, or the common cold if these are associated with the ear infection.

ECZEMA

Eczema, also referred to as *atopic dermatitis*, is one of the most common of childhood complaints. It is characterized by an itchy, red, inflamed rash that commonly appears around the ears, backs of the knees, elbows, forearms, or virtually anywhere. The rash may be weepy and wet and might ooze with scratching. Often, it will appear as small bubbles under the skin. The rash can also be

**External Conditions
That Aggravate Eczema**

- Sweating
- Heat
- Wool (use cotton next to the skin)
- Water and chlorinated water
- Soaps, detergents, perfumes
- Scratching
- Cold weather

dry, red, scaly, and cracked, which may cause thickening of the skin. Both wet and dry eczema cause itching. If the child scratches the rash, he could get a secondary bacterial infection. If your child scratches at night while asleep have him or her wear pajamas, socks, or gloves while sleeping. When the eczema occurs on the buttocks of an infant, the chance of getting a secondary fungal infection increases.

Eczema is an allergic response to an allergen, many times food-related or due to a substance the skin comes in contact with, such as a soap, detergent, metal, or chemical. Infants who get eczema most often get it from a food source in the breast milk or formula or with food introduction. The rash often appears around the mouth, rectum, neck, buttocks, or in the leg and arm creases. This is a sign that there is a malfunction of the digestive system. Prior to birth, the baby receives its nourishment from the mother and its own digestive system is unused. Once the child is born, one of its biggest challenges is to digest foods. The digestive system is not prepared to digest all types of foods, and problems may arise. It is not uncommon to see infantile eczema followed in later years by asthma or hay fever.

Eczema may be triggered by many foods, external irritants, or emotional factors. Common foods include baby formula (both cow and soy), dairy, eggs, wheat, corn, soy, and citrus. Often, an emotional upset, anxiety, or stress will trigger the onset of childhood eczema. This is the body saying that all is not right, and the child is disturbed by the problem or situation. Common triggers are anxiety about school, moving, family separation, or divorce.

If a child has a family history of eczema, asthma, or hay fever, there is a stronger chance that the child will develop eczema. Breast-feeding can help to avoid digestive irritation and strengthen the immune system. I recommend at least six months of breast-feeding for babies with a strong allergic family history.

Treatments

General treatment of the eczema should address the underlying causes of the condition. Identifying offending foods and substances, addressing allergic tendency, and building up the digestive and immune systems should be part of the plan. (See Part II, Working with the Young Immune System, starting on page 19.)

Supplementation

- Essential fatty acids in the form of raw vegetable oils, flaxseed oil, and cod liver oil are highly recommended. Use these daily at a dose of 1 to 3 teaspoons a day, for 6 to 12 months.
- Give zinc, 10 to 30 milligrams, daily.
- Bioflavonoids, 100 to 500 milligrams, daily, should be administered.
- Acidophilus powder, ½ to 1 teaspoon, daily, will help combat eczema.

Also, eat a diet high in these nutrients. (See Part III, Nutrition for Infants and Children, starting on page 37.)

Herbal Treatments

Choose herbs that can correct the imbalance of the digestive, immune, and nervous systems.

- Nourishing, alterative herbs that support waste removal from the body, as well as lymphatic and liver cleansing, can be used as teas taken several times a day for several months. Choose herbs such as burdock root, calendula flowers, cleavers, dandelion, nettles, and red clover.
- Adrenal-supporting herbs such as ashwagandha, licorice, Siberian ginseng, and wild yam may be included to support the body's anti-inflammatory process.
- Immune-building herbs like astragalus, calendula, echinacea, and reishi mushroom work to correct the body's imbalance.
- Nervines and relaxants such as chamomile, lavender flowers, lemon balm, linden flowers, oats, and skullcap should be included when anxiety or stress has a role in the eczema picture. Also use in baths and skin creams.

Topical

Herbal preparations such as washes, creams, oils, or salves can be helpful in resolving inflammation, encouraging the skin to heal, moistening the skin, and restoring normal skin function. If the skin is inflamed use compresses or a wash of chamomile flowers, yarrow flowers, and chickweed. Burdock root decoction can also be used. Use creams or salves with calendula, chamomile, comfrey root, lavender flowers, plantain leaf, or yarrow flowers to moisten the skin, reduce inflammation, and encourage skin healing. If the eczema is wet and weepy, use creams; if it is dry and scaly, use a salve.

Chamomile/Yarrow Eczema Cream
1 2/3 oz. coconut oil
2/3 oz. almond oil
1 oz. rose water
10 drops each of the essential oils of chamomile and yarrow flowers

Weigh all ingredients. Put the oils into a double boiler and stir until melted. While oil mixture is heating, gently heat the flower water. When both are ready, take them off the heat and start adding the rose water a few drops at a time to the oil mixture while beating with a whisk. Beat just until all the water has been absorbed, and then mix in the essential oils. Put into jars and leave in a cool place to set.

FEVER

Fever, a common symptom associated with many childhood illnesses and infections, is often feared by parents and thus suppressive treatments are used too frequently. This may not always be the most beneficial measure for the child. Fever is a defense mechanism the body uses to fight infections. Fever in itself is not the disease. A rise in body temperature occurs in response to substances released by the bacteria or viruses that are being destroyed by the immune system. The rise in temperature enhances the ability of the immune system to destroy the infection, inhibits the reproduction of viruses and bacteria, and aids the body in getting rid of the toxins and waste products. Thus, the fever can be looked at as a strong and vital sign that the immune system is doing its job. As long as the child's immune system is healthy, most illnesses accompanied by fever are easily overcome.

For a small minority of children, high fever can cause febrile seizures. These are seldom associated with brain damage although they can be frightening to the parent. They are most common in babies and children up to the age of three and seldom occur after the age of five.

The first signs of fever are often irritability, grumpiness, and the desire to be close to the parent. The face and cheeks are flushed and warm to the touch. The child may feel either too hot or too cool and the appetite is reduced. In babies and toddlers, the onset is often sudden, occurring over a few hours. With children, the degree of fever may not reflect the severity of the disease process. Extremes of temperature may occur without relation to the significance of the infection. A small infant may have a very serious illness with normal temperatures, whereas a two- to five-year-old child may have a fever above 104°F with a minor respiratory infection. In children over eight years old, temperature response is similar to adults.

Treatments

Fever producing a temperature of 101°F or lower can be managed by giving plenty of fluids such as water, diluted fruit juices, and herbal teas that support the fever and the immune system and avoid dehydration. Warm fluids will help to encourage sweating. Often, it is best with such a low temperature to let the body do its own work. If the fever persists or rises over 101°F, other treatments may be engaged to manage the fever: giving herbs that promote sweating and cooling of the body, using tepid sponge baths with herbal infusions, and cleansing the body with herbal enemas.

Consult your doctor if:

- The temperature is higher that 103°F and it does not respond to fever-reducing treatments.
- The child acts confused or loses consciousness.
- The child has rolling of the eyes or body twitching.
- The infant is under six weeks old.
- There is persistent fever accompanied by headache and stiff neck.

When treating a fever, keep food to a minimum. Most children naturally have no appetite while experiencing a fever, and the appetite often returns as the fever resolves and the temperature returns to normal. While the body is fighting infection with a fever, it cannot spare the energy to digest food. Taking regular amounts of food during a fever may interrupt the body's ability to deal with the fever. It is more important to keep the child hydrated with fluids. Diluted fruit juices, vegetable juices, vegetable broths, miso broth, honey and lemon water, and herbal teas will provide enough nourishment for the few days of fever. As the fever abates, the appetite will return and foods can be introduced once again.

Babies, between six weeks and six months old, with fevers often respond to a warm herbal enema of catnip and fennel seed. This clears out the bowels, and the herb is absorbed into the body through the colon wall. Use a bulb syringe with a warm infusion of herbs. Oil the tip of the bulb with olive oil and place into the rectum one-half inch. Gently squeeze the bulb to release the tea. Place the baby on a towel, as the tea will come back out in a minute or two.

There are many herbs that may be helpful in the management of fevers; however, one must remember that the body produces a fever for a reason and choose the herbs accordingly. Some herbs work to maintain a fever so it will not go too high, others work to support the fever and move it through its course, while others simply suppress the fever.

- Catnip is best as a warm-to-hot tea. Mix it with a pleasant-tasting herb like spearmint or peppermint to hide its bitter flavor. It may also be used as an herbal enema.
- Yarrow may be used as a hot infusion, tincture, warm bath, or with apple cider vinegar as a foot wrap to maintain the fever and keep it from rising too high. For a tea, mix it with peppermint or fennel seed to make it taste more pleasant.
- Elder flowers may also be used as a hot infusion, tincture, or bath to produce sweating, cool the body, and fight the infection. It combines well with catnip and yarrow.
- Meadowsweet helps to promote sweating and acts on the temperature center of the central nervous system to lower the fever.
- Hyssop can be very useful in fevers associated with respiratory infections and cough.
- Chamomile is always a supportive addition to any fever remedy. It aids in reducing the fever, stimulates the immune response, and helps the child to relax, rest, and sleep.
- Garlic rubbed on the feet with a little olive oil before bed will act slowly during the night to stabilize the fever.

Fever Formula

One of my favorite blends for fever, which I use as a tea, tincture, or bath, is a combination of:

1 part elder flowers
1 part linden flowers

1 part peppermint
½ part catnip
½ part yarrow flowers

I often sweeten the tea with a little fruit juice or honey.
Have the child sip it as warm as possible. Up to 1 cup can
be given every 2 hours. As a tincture, use a dose of 10 to 30
drops in a little warm water every 2 hours. For a bath,
make a strong infusion and add to the bathtub or sponge
the child with the warm tea. Bathe freely as needed to manage the fever.

Essential Oils

Essential oils can be used in two ways when working with fevers.
Some oils such as rosemary, lavender, tea tree, and yarrow work
to promote sweating, encouraging the resolution of the fever.
Other oils can be used to cool the body, lowering the temperature,
and thereby avoiding the risk of febrile seizures. Oils that cool the
body include bergamot, eucalyptus, and peppermint. Use 4 to 6
drops of an oil in a tepid sponge or footbath, or add to a massage
oil and rub on the feet and back of the neck and shoulders.

HAND, FOOT, AND MOUTH DISEASE

Hand, foot, and mouth disease is a common contagious illness
caused by the Coxsackie virus. The disease is prevalent during
warm weather, and the average incubation period is three to five
days. It is transmitted by mouth-to-mouth contact or by the oral-
fecal route. It is commonly seen in day-care centers and
preschools.

The illness is characterized by blisters and sores in the mouth
(cheeks, tongue, lips, throat) plus small, clear blisters on the fin-

gers, hands, feet, and toes. Fever may be absent, low, or high. The illness lasts for three to five days. If an infant gets this disease, contact your doctor.

Treatments

Internal

- Support the immune system with immune-enhancing herbs and help to resolve the infection with antiviral herbs such as licorice, lemon balm, echinacea, usnea, astragalus, and garlic.

  With a fever, combine with linden flowers, yarrow flowers, catnip, meadowsweet, or elder flowers. A good combination might be:
  1 part echinacea tincture
  1 part garlic syrup
  1 part astragalus root glycerite
  1 part licorice tincture
  ½ part ginger syrup
  ½ part burdock tincture

  Give ½ to 1 teaspoon, 4 times a day. This same formula can be made as an infusion and sweetened with honey.

- Give immune-supporting vitamins and minerals in the following doses: vitamin C, 200 to 500 milligrams, 3 times a day; zinc, 10 to 15 milligrams, daily; and bioflavonoids, 100 to 500 milligrams, daily.
- Give lots of fluids; have the child sip water, diluted fruit juice, or herbal teas or punches frequently. This keeps the throat moist, the body hydrated, and checks the fever.

Herbal popsicles made from medicinal herbs and fruit juice provide a way to offer fluids and cool the discomfort in the throat and mouth. Use teas that are made from chamomile, elder flowers, spearmint, licorice, lemon balm, wintergreen, willow, ginger, and linden flowers.

External

Use hand and footbaths made from herbal infusions and decoctions to dry up the blisters and heal the skin. Combine 2 or 3 of the following herbs: burdock root, yarrow flowers, comfrey leaf, peppermint, calendula flowers, witch hazel bark, or raspberry leaf. The same herbs can be used to make an herbal mouthwash to treat the blisters in the mouth.

HAY FEVER

Hay fever is an allergic reaction of the membranes of the nose and sinuses to inhaled substances. When it occurs only during a particular time of the year or seasonally, hay fever is usually due to pollens carried in the air. Pollens of trees, grasses, and flowering weeds are the most common allergens. When the hay fever occurs year-round or perennially, it may be due to animal dander, feathers, dust, or mold. Cat, dog, horse, and cow danders are most common; occasionally the culprits are mice, hamsters, guinea pigs, or gerbils. Many foods contain pollens and may also contribute to the reaction.

The irritation of the mucous membranes causes nasal congestion, sneezing, clear nasal discharge, itchy nose, watery itchy eyes, and headache. The ears feel full and blocked, are sometimes painful, and hearing may be diminished due to fluid in the ear.

The membranes become hypersensitive and are more likely to react to new allergens. For instance, a child may get hay fever reactions from animal dander and a few years later start to get it in response to seasonal pollens due to breakdown in the membranes.

Hay fever rarely occurs in children younger than five years old and commonly affects teens and young adults. Hay fever is often seen in children with an allergic history or a family history of allergy, asthma, or ezcema. These children need to have the immune system built up and the allergic immune response stabilized. This will diminish the oversusceptiblity of the immune system and respiratory system to pollens, danders, dusts, and molds. Sugar consumption has an inhibiting effect on the immune system. Thus, it can increase the risk of allergies. Avoiding sugars, sweets, corn syrup, large amounts of fruit juices, and other processed sugars can be very effective in resolving hay fever. Avoiding wheat and wheat products such as breads, cereals, flours, and pasta during seasonal episodes of hay fever caused by pollens will lighten the immune system's load so it can cope with the airborne pollen. Wheat is a member of the grass family and is a high source of dietary pollens. Intolerance to milk and milk products will predispose the child to hay fever and should also be avoided during these episodes.

Treatments

- Keeping the house, particularly the bedroom, well-vacuumed and dry will help minimize irritation. Use non-allergenic pillows, avoid feather or foam (molds love to grow here), use an air purifier or dehumidifier, and change heating duct filters regularly to keep the air free of irritants.
- Eliminate food allergens and foods that burden the immune response. Avoid hydrogenated fats and fried foods to limit the inflammatory reaction of the immune system. Increase

fresh vegetables and fruits such as berries, grapes, plums, and cherries.

- Herbal remedies that quiet the allergic reaction, such as chamomile flowers, eyebright, ephedra, fenugreek seeds, garlic, nettles, and ginger, can be combined with herbs that decongest the membranes, such as cayenne, elder flowers, fenugreek seed, garlic, or horseradish and herbs that strengthen the mucous membranes, such as elder flowers, eyebright, ribwort, or red clover blossoms. These may be used as teas, tinctures, capsules, or syrups. Here are a few combinations I recommend.

Combine fenugreek seed and elder flower tea with a dash of ginger. Take hot several times a day to decongest and open the sinus passages.

Mix 2 ounces of garlic syrup with ½ ounce of eyebright tincture and ¼ ounce each of horseradish tincture and ginger syrup. Take ½ to 1 teaspoon, 3 or 4 times a day.

Ephedra is specific for hay fever, opening up the respiratory passages, and reducing the reaction. It should be used in small doses and not at night, as it may disturb sleep. Use a combination of 1 part eyebright and nettles to ½ part ephedra and goldenseal. Give 30 to 60 drops, 4 to 5 times a day.

Eyebright, elder flowers, ground ivy, or ribwort can be used if the secretions are copious. They will help to dry the membranes and reduce the overproduction of mucus.

Chamomile and lavender flowers used as an herbal steam or put in a hot bath will shrink the membranes and reduce the inflammation. They may be used as infusions or as essential oils.

Lavaging the nasal passages with warm saline water and equal parts of goldenseal/eyebright tea will reduce swelling and congestion.

HEAD LICE

These tiny parasites, less than one-eighth of an inch long, are grayish white, transparent creatures with six legs. They live only on humans, never on pets. They pass from person to person by close contact, hats, hairbrushes, and combs. Head lice can live away from the body for up to twenty-four hours hiding in pillows, sheets, towels, and clothing. They live on or close to the scalp where they bite and suck blood. They are often hard to see and are most easily found at the hairline on the back of the neck. The females lay eggs, or nits, which stick to the hair and look like little white specks but will not brush out. The nits hatch in about eight days and each louse lives about five weeks.

Head lice cause itching of the scalp and sometimes a red, scaly rash on the back of the neck at the hairline. Due to scratching, sores on the scalp may occur. If severe, the sores may become infected. The lymph nodes at the base of the skull may enlarge.

Treatments

- Clean combs, hairbrushes, hats, bed linen, and towels.
- Use a combination of 4 ounces of olive oil mixed with 3 teaspoons of an essential oil mix. Choose several of the following: tea tree, eucalyptus, rosemary, lavender, hyssop, or pennyroyal. Apply the aromatic oil to the scalp and hair thoroughly. Cover with a shower cap and leave on until morning. In the morning, use a nit comb to comb through the hair, then wash out the oil with a tea tree oil shampoo

and rinse with a tea of rosemary and sage. Do not rinse out. Comb the hair again with the nit comb. Repeat each night for 1 week and once a week after that for 3 weeks.

- Use 2 or 3 drops of rosemary or lavender oil rubbed into the hairbrush and brushed through the hair. This will help to deter lice.
- Blow dry hair with a hair dryer 5 to 10 minutes a day, for 7 to 10 days. This helps to kill the nits as well as the adult lice.

HEADACHES

Headaches are commonly associated with fever, food allergy, constipation, liver congestion, upper respiratory infection, and emotional upsets such as fear, anxiety, worry, and sadness. Less commonly, they are associated with head trauma, tumor, meningitis, and intracranial bleeding.

Food intolerance or allergic reactions are often associated with chronic headaches. Finding and eliminating the offending foods is important. (See Food Allergy, page 31.) Migraine headaches are often associated with trigger foods such as chocolate, cheese, citrus, or fermented foods as well as to food allergies. Children who have migraine headaches often have a strong family history of migraines or allergic syndromes. The headache is often more one-sided and is generally accompanied by nausea and vomiting and may be preceded by an aura or visual disturbances. A migraine may last for hours.

Headaches associated with constipation may also be due to food intolerance, poor digestive function, and tension. Increasing the child's water intake is often a key, along with treating the digestion. (See Constipation, page 100.) If the headache is due to muscle tension or stress and worry, treat with herbal relaxants like crampbark, catnip, or lemon balm and nervines like hops, oats, and skullcap to reduce muscle tension and stress.

Treatments

- Be sure to treat the underlying cause of the headaches as discussed in the previous section. Using herbal muscle relaxants, pain relievers, and nervines to reduce the pain and discomfort can be helpful for relieving the symptoms. Use herbs in teas, baths, body rubs, tinctures, and essential oils.
- Herbal muscle relaxants aid in reducing the tension of the muscles, blood vessels, and soft tissue. They can relieve constrictive headaches due to muscle spasm or poor blood flow. Herbs such as crampbark, catnip, lavender flowers, lemon balm, and small amounts of lobelia can be used.
- Herbal pain relievers such as meadowsweet, willow bark, and wintergreen diminish the pain and discomfort of the headache. These all make pleasant teas or can be used as tinctures. Wintergreen as a body rub will help to reduce muscle spasm and pain.
- Herbal nervines aid in relaxing the nervous system and in reducing tension in the body. Many of these plants also have a relaxing effect on the body tissues. Use the following herbs in teas, tinctures, baths, or oils: chamomile, hops, lemon balm, lavender, linden flowers, oatgrass, skullcap, and passionflower.

Topical Headache Rub

Mix together in a 2-ounce amber bottle:

½ oz. of lobelia oil
½ oz. of St. John's wort oil
½ oz. of crampbark tincture

¼ oz. of wintergreen essential oil

¼ oz. of lavender essential oil

Shake well before using, as contents will separate when stored. Rub on the forehead and back of the neck as needed.

HIVES

Hives (or urticaria), an allergic reaction of the skin, are red, itchy, raised welts that range from one-quarter inch to several inches in size. The welts can appear on any part of the body and change rapidly in appearance. Many things can cause a hive reaction including foods, colorings, preservatives, prescription medicines, soaps, sun, heat, any skin contactants, bug bites, animals, parasite infections, emotional stress, and many more. Common foods that may cause hives include citrus fruits, chocolate, peanut butter, nuts, shellfish, tomatoes, berries, and sweets.

Treatments

It is important to identify the allergen causing the hives and to avoid exposure. Look over the activities and what has been eaten over the hours preceding the onset of hives. Conventional treatments include oral antihistamines. Many natural remedies have antihistamine activity.

- Vitamin C in the buffered powdered form can be given at a dose of 200 to 500 milligrams, 4 times a day, to stop the allergic reaction.
- Quercetin, a bioflavonoid that inhibits the release of histamine, can be given at 250 to 500 milligrams, 4 times a day. Nettles can be given to slow the allergic response and

diminish itchiness of the skin. Use in the freeze-dried capsule form, 1 or 2 capsules every 2 hours. Drinking nettle tea
and washing the area with a strong tea is also helpful.

- A warm herbal bath is a great way to relieve the discomfort
and inflammation of the reaction. Make an infusion from a
mixture of chickweed, comfrey, and burdock. Add to a
warm bath and let the child soak for 20 to 30 minutes.

HYPERACTIVITY

Hyperactivity, also known as attention deficit/hyperactivity disorder (ADHD), can affect children of all ages as well as adults.
It has been estimated that 10 percent of boys and 3 percent of
girls between the ages of four and eleven are afflicted. This is a
very real disorder yet the term can be used too freely, and incor-
rectly labeling a child with ADHD can be a terrible error. Children are active and energetic, don't always listen or sit still, and
can be disruptive. Not all children learn in the typical environment, and often, the classroom structure is not a productive environment. Being sure about the diagnosis before using the term is
very important. The main features of ADHD are difficulty getting things done and focusing on tasks, short attention span,
impulsiveness, difficulty getting along with other children and
adults, hyperactivity, and learning and behavioral problems.
These children are often above-average intellectually, have low
self-esteem, and are sad.

Hyperactivity may be related to heavy-metal toxicity, such as
lead poisoning; visual or hearing problems; mineral deficiency;
seizures; and prenatal alcohol or drug exposure. These should be
ruled out before using the label ADHD. The exact causes of
ADHD are unknown but among them may be genetic factors,
chemical imbalance, injury at birth, neonatal disease, and brain

or nervous system defects. One factor that many clinicians agree on is that lifestyle aspects can reduce behavioral problems with these children, even if the cause is not clear.

Early diagnosis, intervention, and treatment for these children are important and may affect their lives as adults, as there is a greater risk that children suffering from ADHD will suffer from depression, restlessness, or have substance abuse problems.

Treatments

Lifestyle Considerations

- Set a stable routine for the child's day, one that minimizes stimulation, is organized, and has specific mealtimes and bedtimes.
- Limit or avoid TV and video games or get them out of the house all together.
- Give the child simple, quickly accomplished tasks and give positive reinforcement when they are completed.
- Regular exercise, playing outdoors, yoga, tai chi, or martial arts are excellent ways to encourage better concentration and higher self-esteem.
- Seek the help of a counselor for the child and family.

Dietary Recommendations

- Encourage a whole-food diet with as many organic foods as possible and foods high in complex carbohydrates and proteins. Include a variety of foods, raw oils, organic live yogurt (if no dairy allergy), and lots of good water.
- Avoid processed junk food, refined carbohydrates, sugars, all soda pop, food additives, food colorings, and food preservatives. Reduction of the following foods has been shown to reduce behavioral and sleep problems: artificial

food colorings, additives, preservatives, monosodium gluta-
mate (MSG), chocolate, caffeine, and sugar. The following
food additives should be completely avoided: tartrazine, all
yellow dyes, benzoic acid, FCF, carmolic acid, sulfur dioxide, caramel, sodium nitrate, sodium benzoate, BHT, BHA,
potassium nitrate, Red 2G, and blue dyes.

- Foods high in salicylates have been linked to hyperactivity.
  Salicylates are found in many fruits, vegetables, herbs, and
  spices and can be tricky to eliminate entirely. Here is a list
  of foods known to be high in salicylates: almonds, peanuts,
  tomatoes, peas, cucumbers, pickles, green peppers, honey,
  apples, bananas, rasberries, peaches, plums, prunes, grapes,
  raisins, peppermint, oranges, and spices like clove, cinnamon, and curry. Wintergreen, willow bark, and meadowsweet are also high in salicylates.
- Identify and treat any underlying food allergies. (See Part II,
  Working with the Young Immune System, starting on page 19.)

Supplementation

- DHA, docosahexanoic acid, is an essential fatty acid that is
  found in high concentrations in the brain and is essential
  for normal neurological development in infants. There is
  some speculation that children with ADHD have lower levels of this essential fatty acid. The dose is 200 to 250 milligrams, daily.
- Administer vitamin B complex with at least 100 milligrams
  of B6 in a balance of all the other B vitamins, including
  choline.
- Give magnesium citrate, 150 milligrams to 200 milligrams,
  daily. Please note that some children can get soft or loose
  stool from magnesium supplementation. If this occurs, cut
  the dose in half.

- Glycine, an amino acid, has a calming effect on the nervous system and the brain. Give ½ teaspoon in diluted, clear fruit juice in the morning and evening.
- Chromium, 100 micrograms, 2 times a day before meals in liquid form, will stabilize blood sugar metabolism.
- Serine is an amino acid that has a blood-sugar regulating effect in the body and can inhibit overstimulation of the adrenal gland by the hypothalamus-pituitary axis. In other words, it helps to quiet the body and mind. Five-hundred milligrams given at dinner and bedtime will produce a deeper and more restful sleep.

Herbal Treatments

- Nervine herbs have been traditionally used in the treatment of hyperactivity. There are a number of herbs that may be used for this purpose, but I would like to mention a few in particular: wild oat (*Avena sativa*) is calming, restoring, relaxing, and strengthening to the nervous system and tissue; lemon balm (*Melissa officinalis*) acts to calm nervous irritability, sensitivity, and excitement, and its warm, lemony scent enhances mood and sleep; passionflower (*Passiflora incarnata*) contains several compounds that have mild calming effects, mood-enhancing action, and aid in improving concentration. Last, I need to mention skullcap (*Scutellaria* spp.) for its strong tonifying effect on the nervous system and its ability to relax muscle and nerve agitation and to calm the mind. Several of these herbs are often mixed together.
- Gotu kola is a helpful herb for ADHD children, as it has demonstrated an ability to enhance mental functions, such as concentration, memory, and alertness, while also having a mild anti-anxiety and relaxing effect.

- Melissa Supreme for Children (available from Gaia Herbs) is a blend of lemon balm, chamomile flowers, passion-flower, skullcap, and wild oat. Gotu kola and Irish moss is a specific formula for improving concentration. Age-related doses are on the bottle.
- A combination of skullcap, wild oats, and ginger makes a spicy-tasting formula to help with ADHD. Give 5 drops in juice for 3- to 5-year-olds and 10 drops to 6- to 12-year-olds in water or juice, 3 or 4 times a day.
- Passionflower/lemon balm formula (available from Gaia Herbs) is a great formula with a more relaxing, sedating effect, and it can be used at night to calm the mind, nerves, and body. Use as directed.
- Adaptogen herbs such as *Eleutherococcus senticosus* and *Withania somnifera* help to strengthen the body by building up the nervous system and aiding the body's ability to deal with the effects of stress. *Withania* has the reputation for promoting learning and memory recollection. These herbs are meant to be taken over time, acting as tonics. A combination of the two in equal parts of a tincture should be given daily. The dose for a 2- to 4-year-old would be ¼ teaspoon, ½ teaspoon for a 5- to 8-year-old, and 1 teaspoon for a 9- to 13-year-old.

IMPETIGO

Impetigo is a highly contagious staphylococcus bacterial infection of the skin that is commonly found around the lips, chin, nose, and ears. It typically starts as fragile blisters that contain a yellowish fluid. They break open and leave highly infectious, weepy sores. The sores dry and form a yellowish, crusted scab.

Sometimes impetigo comes as a secondary infection to eczema, hives, diaper rash, or bug bites.

It is important to prevent spreading this disease to other parts of the body or to other people. To discourage the child from scratching the sores, use loose gauze coverings. Keep the child's washcloths, towels, and bed linens separate from other family member's and wash the hands frequently and well.

Treatments

- Wash the affected area several times a day with calendula or tea tree soap and warm water; pat dry with a paper towel.
- Apply an herbal skin wash made from echinacea, goldenseal, calendula flowers, and lavender flowers to the skin several times a day.
- Make an herbal lotion made from ½ ounce each of lavender, echinacea, myrrh, and calendula tinctures mixed with 2 ounces of water. Apply several times a day with cotton balls.
- Use a few drops of lavender essential oil in a cream or salve base and apply to the sores after washing.
- The following formula can be given as a tea: 1 cup, 3 times a day, or as a tincture, 60 drops, 4 times a day.
- Mix 1 part each of echinacea, usnea, and red clover with ½ part each of peppermint and ginger.

INFLUENZA

Influenza is a highly contagious, respiratory infection that is caused by the influenza A or B virus. It is transmitted by droplets from the nose and throat discharge of infected people. It has a short incubation period of one to three days.

Symptoms include sudden chills, fever ranging from 102°F to 105°F, flushing, headache, sore throat, hacking cough, redness of the eyes, and pains in the back and limbs. In young children vomiting and diarrhea may occur. The fever lasts three to four days and is followed by a few days of weakness and fatigue. During this period, the child is more vulnerable to other illness. The fever associated with influenza often peaks in two cycles. It will be elevated for a few days, normal for a day, and elevated again for a few days.

Secondary bacterial complications are common, and their presence is suggested by the return of high fever after the third or fourth day of normal temperature; progressive worsening of cough, changing to loose and productive; yellowish nasal discharge; pus in the eyes; and ear infection. Secondary bacterial infections can be severe due to the already compromised state of the immune defenses from the viral infection. Recovery can often take several weeks.

Treatments

Internal

- Support the immune system with immune-enhancing herbs and help to resolve the infection with antiviral herbs such as licorice, lemon balm, echinacea, usnea, astragalus, and garlic. For the fever, combine with linden flowers, yarrow flowers, catnip, meadowsweet, or elder flowers.

Flu Combination
1 part echinacea tincture
1 part garlic syrup

1 part astragalus root glycerite
1 part licorice tincture
1 part lemon balm tincture or glycerite
1 part linden flowers tincture
½ part ginger syrup
½ part elder flowers tincture

Give ½ to 1 teaspoon, 4 times a day. This same formula can be made as an infusion and sweetened with honey.

- Give immune-supporting vitamins and minerals in the following doses: vitamin C, 200 to 500 milligrams, 3 times a day; zinc, 10 to 15 milligrams, daily; and bioflavonoids, 100 to 500 milligrams, daily.
- Give lots of fluids; have the child sip water, diluted fruit juice, or herbal teas or punches frequently. This keeps the throat moist, the body hydrated, and checks the fever.
- Herbal popsicles made from medicinal herbs and fruit juice is a good way to offer fluids and cool the discomfort in the throat and mouth. Use teas made from cleavers, elder flowers, spearmint, licorice, lemon balm, wintergreen, red clover, ginger, and linden flowers.

External

- Use herbal baths and washes made from infusions of elder flowers, yarrow flowers, rosemary, and peppermint to cool the fever.
- Use herbal chest rubs on the back and chest to quiet the cough and relax breathing. (See Recipes and Remedies for Infants and Children, starting on page 265.)
- Use a few drops of essential oils on a cotton ball and place in the tray of a vaporizer where the steam is released.

Choose from eucalyptus, rosemary, thyme, lavender, or tea tree oil.

- At the first sign of illness, use a few drops of essential oil of eucalyptus, tea tree, or lavender in a hot bath for 10 minutes to produce sweating, followed by a night of sleep. This will attack the virus and stimulate the immune response.

INSECT BITES

The bites or stings of most insects are minor annoyances to most children. However, bees and wasps can cause an acute and severe allergic reaction in some children, marked by hives, asthma, and collapse. Flying insects only bite exposed skin; crawling insects bite anywhere and often in groups. Flea bites tend to be concentrated around the lower leg and ankle. Ticks remain attached to the skin for long periods while biting and resemble small, plump raisins as they swell. Bites from deer ticks can be serious and might lead to Lyme disease, which is caused by a bacteria transmitted by the tick. See your doctor if your child has had a tick bite and presents with a round, red skin lesion three to thirty-two days later, accompanied with flulike symptoms, headache, or stiff neck. Common areas for the lesions are the thighs, buttocks, and underarms.

Treatments

- Make a fresh poultice of plantain leaves, sliced onion, or raw grated potato. (See Making Herbal Preparations, starting on page 259.) Apply for 10 minutes. It will draw out the poison and relieve itching.
- Make a compress of distilled witch hazel with a few drops of lavender oil. This can also be used as a lotion for larger areas around bites.

- Herbal smudges made from burning herbs help to repel insects. Try using herbs like sage, rosemary, wormwood, cedar, or eucalyptus. Place a small amount of dry herb on a bit of charcoal in a small dish or shell and burn slowly.

Bug Repellent
Mix together 15 drops each of the essential oils lavender, citronella, eucalyptus, and pennyroyal with 1 ounce of almond or olive oil. Use on clothing or directly on the skin.

LARYNGITIS

Laryngitis is an inflammation of the voice box (larynx). Laryngitis is almost always caused by a respiratory virus. Symptoms of largyngitis include a hoarse voice, dry hacking cough, scratchy throat, and a low-grade fever (101°F or lower). Laryngitis lasts from one to fourteen days. If the child presents with associated breathing difficulties, consult your doctor.

Treatments

- Give immune-supporting vitamins and minerals, use an immune-supportive diet, and take lots of warm liquids. (See Part II, Working with the Young Immune System, starting on page 19.)
- Using a vaporizor in the room where the child sleeps will keep the air moist. If you put a cotton ball saturated with lavender or rosemary oil near the opening that releases the steam, it will disperse the oil into the air and into the child's respiratory system, moistening the throat and purifying the air.
- Give warm herbal teas made from licorice, lemon balm, chamomile, thyme, echinacea, elder flowers, or red clover.

- Zinc or herbal aromatic throat lozenges taken regularly during the day make a good local treatment. Check your health food store.
- Apply a warm neck compress 2 times a day, for 20 minutes. (See instructions for Mullein/Lobelia Neck Wrap and Carrot Poultice on page 267.)

Herbal Compound for Laryngitis
½ oz. echinacea tincture
½ oz. garlic syrup
½ oz. lemon balm tincture
¼ oz. catnip tincture
¼ oz. cleavers glycerite
¼ oz. cinnamon tincture

Mix in a 2-ounce amber bottle and give ½ teaspoon, every 2 hours.

MEASLES

This infectious childhood disease is highly contagious, passing from child to child by an airborne or droplet-borne virus. The incubation period for measles is ten to twelve days, and it can be passed on from the fifth day of incubation through the first few days of the rash. The disease usually starts as a cold with a fever, cough, runny nose, and conjunctivitis. There may be white spots on the inside lining of the cheek known as Koplik's spots, which look very much like little grains of salt surrounded by red rims. After three or four days, the fever rises to 104°F or 105°F and is accompanied by a rash. The rash starts as flat, reddish spots appearing first behind the ears, under the arms, and on the neck and face. As more spots appear, they merge together, forming red patches. The rash quickly spreads over the back, abdomen, and head, and less often to the legs and arms. Other symptoms that can occur include nausea, vomiting, diarrhea, abdominal pain, and swollen lymph nodes in the neck and underarms. Once the rash has fully erupted, the fever breaks and the child improves. Some children suffer other complications from measles. Common ones are middle ear infection, pneumonia, bronchitis, or, rarely, encephalitis. If a child becomes sick again or has a rise in fever ten days after the measles are gone, call your doctor.

Once a child has had measles, he or she has lifelong immunity. A breast-feeding baby will have immunity if the mother does for the first six months of life. Many parents choose to immunize their children against measles. Immunized children can be contagious just after receiving the live vaccine, and, if they do contact measle virus, they can still be contagious even though they do not get the disease.

Treatments

Internal

- To help resolve the infection give antivirals such as licorice, lemon balm, echinacea, and garlic. For the fever combine with catnip, yarrow flowers, meadowsweet, linden flowers, or elder flowers. To improve lymphatic drainage and aid release of toxins from the skin, use cleavers, calendula, burdock, or peppermint. For irritability and restlessness, include skullcap, chamomile, lavender, or catnip.

  Measles Formula
  1 part echinacea tincture or glycerite
  1 part garlic syrup
  1 part peppermint tincture

1 part lemon balm tincture or glycerite
1 part cleavers glycerite
1 part burdock root tincture
1 part skullcap glycerite
½ part catnip tincture
½ part elder flowers tincture

Give ½ to 1 teaspoon, 4 times a day. Using dried herbs, this same formula can be made as an infusion and sweetened with honey. (See Making Herbal Preparations, starting on page 259.)

- Give immune-supporting vitamins and minerals in the following doses: vitamin C, 200 to 500 milligrams, 3 times a day; zinc, 10 milligrams, daily; bioflavonoids, 100 to 500 milligrams, daily; and lysine, 500 milligrams, 1 or 2 times daily, as an antiviral.
- Give lots of fluids; the child should sip water, diluted fruit juice, or herbal teas or punches, frequently. This keeps the throat moist and checks the fever. Avoid solid foods when the fever is high; give soups and juices instead.
- Herbal popsicles made from medicinal herbs and fruit juice are a good way to offer fluids and cool the discomfort in the throat and mouth. Use teas made from chamomile, cleavers, elder flowers, spearmint, licorice, lemon balm, wintergreen, red clover, and linden flowers. (See Making Herbal Preparations, starting on page 259.)

External

- Use tepid herbal baths or washes to aid the skin in clearing the rash. Use infusions made from chamomile, yarrow flowers, burdock root, calendula flowers, red clover blossoms, or lavender flowers.

- If the eyes become inflamed and sore use herbal eye compresses made from cooled infusions of calendula, chamomile, marshmallow root, or eyebright.

MOTION SICKNESS

Car, air, or seasickness are forms of motion sickness. A motion-sick child becomes nauseated, pale, anxious, and sweaty and may vomit. The child is not able to control the sickness, and it can be very unpleasant for him or her.

Treatments

- Ginger is one of the most effective herbal remedies for motion sickness. It can be used an hour before traveling and taken in small doses while traveling. I prefer to use ginger drops made by adding ¼ ounce of ginger tincture to ¾ ounce of water. The dosage is 10 to 30 drops as needed.
- Herbal teas taken slowly by the teaspoonful can also be helpful; choose herbs like ginger, aniseed, chamomile flowers, and meadowsweet.
- Sea Bands are wrist bracelets that put pressure on acupuncture points to relieve nausea and vomiting. They are available in many health food stores.

MUMPS

Mumps is an infectious viral disease involving swelling of the parotid salivary gland, found in front of, beneath, and behind the ears. The disease is contracted by saliva, with an incubation period of fourteen to twenty-one days. A child can infect others from one to two days before the onset of swelling to three to five days after the swelling has gone. Children who have had mumps have lifelong immunity to the disease.

Typically, a child presents with symptoms of fever (101°F to 104°F), loss of appetite, headache, neck pain, and malaise. One or two days after these symptoms, swelling of the parotid glands appears, usually one side and then the other. Swelling of the glands lasts about a week. Only a swelling of the parotid gland has the ear lobe as its center. Swelling of this gland can make swallowing, eating, and talking uncomfortable and painful. Avoid acidic foods such as vinegar, lemon, tomatoes, or orange juice.

Complications of mumps can sometimes lead to meningitis or encephalitis; call your doctor if neck pain and headache persist after seven to ten days. Mumps in older children or adults may cause swelling of the ovaries, testicles, and pancreas.

Treatments

Internal

- To help resolve the infection give antivirals such as licorice, lemon balm, echinacea, and garlic. For the fever combine with linden flowers, yarrow flowers, meadowsweet, or elder flowers. To improve lymphatic drainage and reduce glandular swelling, add cleavers, calendula, or small amounts of poke root.

Mumps Formula
1 part echinacea tincture
1 part garlic syrup
1 part licorice tincture
1 part lemon balm tincture or glycerite
1 part cleavers glycerite

½ part meadowsweet tincture
½ part calendula flowers succus or juice

Give ½ to 1 teaspoon, 4 times a day. This same formula can be made as an infusion with fresh or dried herbs and sweetened with honey. (See Making Herbal Preparations, starting on page 259.)

- Give immune-supporting vitamins and minerals in the following doses: vitamin C, 200 to 500 milligrams, 3 times a day; zinc, 10 to 15 milligrams, daily; and bioflavonoids, 100 to 500 milligrams, daily.
- Give lots of fluids; have the child sip water, diluted fruit juice, or herbal teas or punches, frequently. This keeps the throat moist and checks the fever.
- Herbal popsicles made from medicinal herbs and fruit juice are a great way to offer fluids and cool the discomfort in the throat and mouth. Freeze teas made from cleavers, elder flowers, spearmint, licorice, lemon balm, wintergreen, red clover, and linden flowers.

External (See Recipes and Remedies for Infants and Children, starting on page 265.)

- Use the diluted essential oils of lavender, rosemary, yarrow, or thyme. Dilute with sweet almond or olive oil.
- Apply the mullein/lobelia neck wrap twice a day for 20 to 30 minutes.
- Apply carrot poultice, 1 to 3 times a day, to reduce swelling and discomfort.
- Warm herbal compresses can be wrapped around the neck and held in place with a towel several times day. Apply a hot water bottle or heating pad for extra warmth. Use wintergreen, lobelia, St. John's wort, lavender, or meadowsweet

for reducing the pain and cleavers, mullein, lobelia, poke root, or wormwood for reducing the swelling.

NOSEBLEEDS

Nosebleeds are as much a part of childhood as bruises and skinned knees. The majority of nosebleeds are caused by the rupturing of small blood vessels in the septum. These tiny blood vessels can be broken due to nose blowing, sneezing, coughing, dryness of the nose, trauma, or nose picking. Nosebleeds can be a sign of allergies or might indicate that the air in the house is too dry or that the heating system is irritating the child. Keeping the air moist with a humidifier, placing a pan of water on the radiator or woodstove, and opening a window in the bedroom while sleeping can help.

Since the nose is connected to the throat there can be vomiting due to blood running down the throat. If the nosebleed occurs after a blow to the head, see your doctor.

Treatments

Have the child sit upright with the mouth open and head held back. Grasp the whole lower half of the nose between the thumb and fingers and compress both sides firmly against the septum of the nose. The nose should be held for ten minutes to allow the blood to clot.

Cold compresses can be applied to the back of the neck or to the nose. Soak the compress in a cool herbal tea such as witch hazel, yarrow flowers, or cayenne pepper.

If nosebleeds occur frequently, the blood vessels can be strengthened by using vitamin C and bioflavonoids in a supplement form. Herbs that also can be used to strengthen the small vessels include blueberry, huckleberry, hawthorne berry, and gingko.

PINWORMS

The pinworm, also known as threadworm or seatworm, is one of the most common parasitic infections affecting humans. It is most common in young children but may affect people of all ages. It is estimated that one out of twenty children is infected each year. Pinworms are one-third- to one-half-inch long, white or yellowish white, with a clear posterior point, and are about as thick as sewing thread. The adult worm lives in the large intestine, and the mature females crawl out of the anus at night to lay thousands of tiny eggs in the perianal skin. Because the egg laying causes intense itching of the perianal area, the usual pathway of infection is from anus to hand to mouth. Once the eggs have been ingested, they live in the intestinal tract and mature in about two to four weeks. The mature worms then live another six to eight weeks. The many tiny eggs contaminate clothing, underwear, sheets, towels, fingernails, and anything else the hands may touch. The eggs are so light that they may float in the air and contaminate most anything they land on. The eggs can stay viable outside a host for up to three weeks.

The symptoms of pinworms may vary from few to several. The most common symptom is rectal itching, particularly at night, from the egg laying. Other symptoms may include interrupted sleep, bad breath, grinding of the teeth, changes in the appetite, changes in stool patterns, abdominal pain, nose picking, lethargy, and bad dreams. Chronic cystitis and vaginitis in little girls can be caused by pinworms.

Checking your child for worms is best done in the first two hours after going to bed. A flashlight may be used to examine the area for worms just after the child has gone to sleep. To check for eggs, get a microscope slide from your health care provider, then press a piece of clear cellophane tape, sticky side down, on to the rectum and perianal folds. Quickly lift the tape and apply the sticky side down on the slide. Place the slide in an envelope to protect it, and take it to your health care provider for microscopic inspection. As pinworms are not active every night, it is best to repeat the test on several different nights.

Typically, young children pick up pinworms at day care or school and bring them into the house. Once pinworms are in the household, everyone is at risk of being infected. Eradication can be difficult, requiring washing of bed linens, towels, pajamas, and underwear with hot water and extra bleach. Scrub all washable toys, toilets, bathtubs, and other high-risk surfaces. Clean and cut fingernails and encourage extra washing of hands and showers. Use a clothes dryer to dry all clothes after washing, as heat and dryness kill the eggs. Repeat these suggestions daily during treatment and for several weeks after.

If you decide to treat with the pharmaceutical drug, Vermox, the dietary and digestive support therapies suggested below are still recommended.

Treatments

- Have your child wear tight-fitting underwear to bed during the treatment. This will help to cut down contamination of the bed sheets. Change them every morning. Apply a salve made with tea tree oil, lavender oil, rosemary oil, or a mixture of all three to the rectum each night to discourage the worms from laying the eggs and to relieve the itching.
- Worms tend to multiple rapidly in children with weak or unhealthy digestive systems. (See Health and the Role of the Digestive System, page 38.) Avoid a high-sugar and simple-

carbohydrate diet, as pinworms seem to thrive on sugars. Include onions, garlic, pumpkin seeds, ginger, cinnamon, and clove in the diet, along with lots of fluids. Avoid a high amount of fruit juices because of their concentrated fruit sugars.

- Puree 6 lemon seeds in 2 ounces of water with ½ teaspoon of stevia powder. Drink on an empty stomach daily for 7 days and repeat in 2 weeks.
- Add 3 to 5 drops of grapefruit seed extract to a small amount of orange juice. Take 2 to 3 times a day for 2 weeks on an empty stomach. Repeat after a 2-week rest period.
- Proteolytic enzymes can be used between meals to fight against the maturing worms. Use bromelain, Zymex II (produced by Standard Process), or a combination formula of several enzymes. Be sure to use between meals, or the enzyme will act only on the food and not on the pinworms.
- Many herbs have anthelmintic properties. They can be given as single remedies or mixed into a compound of several. Some of the most useful anthelmintics include mugwort, garlic, wormwood, clove, black walnut, tansy, sage, and cayenne pepper. Many of these herbs taste bitter and can be mixed with fennel, stevia, or peppermint to improve the flavor. Always give on an empty stomach and at least 2 to 3 times, daily.
- Give pumpkin seeds that are ground up and mixed with grated carrot for breakfast, for 5 to 7 mornings in a row.
- Cina 6c, a homeopathic remedy, is effective in the treatment of pinworms. Use a dose of 2 to 4 pellets, 3 times a day, away from food and drink, for 2 weeks.
- *Lactobacillus g.g.* is an aggressive species of acidophilus that has been shown to be useful in eradicating intestinal parasites. The species is sold under the name Culturelle and is sometimes found in CVS pharmacies. Dose is 1 or 2 cap-

sules, daily, for several weeks. I often recommend doing this along with other anthelmintic treatments.

ROSEOLA

Roseola is an acute viral infectious disease that has a characteristic high fever followed by a rash. This disease occurs almost exclusively in the period from six months to three years of age. The incubation period is seven to fourteen days, and a child has lifelong immunity after one attack. The onset is sudden, with a high fever of 104°F to 106°F. The fever's severity may cause febrile convulsions at the onset. Roseola may be accompanied by a runny nose and swollen lymph glands in the neck. The fever usually persists for three to four days. Often, the child does not seem to be as ill as one would expect with a fever of that degree. The fever resolves suddenly and is followed by the appearance of a splotchy red rash of the trunk, spreading to the arms and neck. The rash lasts a day or two with little or no discomfort. Complications are rare.

Treatments

The most worrisome symptom of this illness is the high fever and the fact that the age group most likely to get this illness is most at risk for febrile seizures. The use of herbal medicines to manage and resolve the fever is an important part of the treatment. Using herbal teas, baths, essential oils, and tinctures will help the body keep the temperature below 103°F and support the immune system in resolving the infection. (See Fever, starting on page 127.)

Herbal teas are easy to give to small children and babies if they have a pleasant taste and are somewhat sweet. Teas can be given to babies in teaspoon doses or with a dropper. They can be taken as frequently as desired until the fever has been resolved. Some of the herbs I recommend follow.

- Catnip is best as a warm-to-hot tea; mix it with a pleasant-tasting herb like spearmint or peppermint to hide its bitter flavor. It may also be used as an herbal enema. (See Making Herbal Preparations, starting on page 259.)
- Yarrow may be used as a hot infusion, tincture, warm bath, or with apple cider vinegar as a foot wrap to maintain the fever and keep it from rising too high. For a tea, mix it with peppermint or fennel seed to make it taste more pleasant.
- Elder flowers also may be used as a hot infusion, tincture, or bath to produce sweating, cool the body, and fight the infection. It combines well with catnip and yarrow.
- Meadowsweet promotes sweating, along with acting on the temperature center of the central nervous system to lower the setting.
- Hyssop can be very useful in fevers associated with respiratory infections and cough.
- Chamomile is always a supportive addition to any fever remedy because it not only aids in reducing the fever but stimulates the immune response and relaxes the child, helping her to rest and sleep.
- Echinacea added to the fever teas or given separately in glycerite or tincture form will help the body fight the virus and move through the illness. Give infants 1 to 2 droppersful of a sweetened decoction of echinacea root or 10 drops of tincture or glycerite diluted with a little water every 2 hours during the fever. Licorice root can be added for taste as well as for its antiviral action.

Fever Combination
One of my favorite blends for fever, which I use as a tea, tincture, or bath, is a combination of:

1 part elder flowers
1 part linden flowers

1 part peppermint
½ part catnip
½ part yarrow flowers

As a tea, use 1 to 2 teaspoons herb mix to 8 ounces of boiling water. Steep for 1 to 2 minutes and strain. Sweeten with a little fruit juice or honey. Have the child sip it as warm as possible. Up to a cup can be given every 2 hours. As a tincture, use 10 to 30 drops in a little warm water, every 2 hours. For a bath make a strong infusion (1 tablespoon to 8 ounces water) and add to the bathtub or sponge the child with the warm tea. Bathe as often as needed to manage the fever.

Healing Bath

This bath will support the immune system in resolving the viral infection, keep the body at a safe temperature, and reduce any discomfort the child is having. Make a strong infusion of 1 teaspoon of each of the following herbs to 2 cups of boiling water and add to the bath: chamomile, hops, lavender flowers, linden flowers, and yarrow flowers.

Essential Oils

Essential oils can be used in two ways when working with fevers. Some oils, such as rosemary, lavender, tea tree, and yarrow, promote sweating, encouraging the resolution of the fever. Other oils can be used to cool the body by lowering the temperature, avoiding the risk of febrile fits. Oils that cool the body include bergamot, eucalyptus, and peppermint. Add 4 to 6 drops of the oil to a tepid sponge or footbath. Or add it to a massage oil and rub on the feet and on the back of the neck and shoulders.

RUBELLA (GERMAN MEASLES)

Rubella, or German measles, is the mildest contagious disease of childhood. It is often so mild that a parent may not know the child has it. It is caused by a specific virus and is spread by droplets, direct contact with the contagious person, or indirectly through contact with contaminated objects. The incubation period is fourteen to twenty-one days, and one attack gives life-long immunity. A child is contagious for the period from seven days prior to onset of the illness until five days after the appearance of the rash.

Rubella often starts with a runny nose, sore throat, and swollen lymph nodes in front of and behind the ears, at the base of the skull, and on the neck. In a day or so, a fine, splotchy, dark pink rash appears on the face and spreads over the rest of the body within twenty-four hours. This generally lasts for three days and may be itchy. There may or may not be a low-grade fever (100°F oral or 101°F rectal), loss of appetite, and malaise.

Although this disease is mild for the child, it can be very dangerous to a fetus if a pregnant woman becomes infected. Rubella during pregnancy may cause miscarriage or congenital problems of the eyes, ears, and heart. If your child has rubella or has had a recent rubella vaccination, have him avoid contact with pregnant women.

Treatments

Illness from rubella is often very mild and the need for treatment is little. Give general immune-supporting, lymphatic, and nutritional herbs to aid the body's defenses. Here's a good herbal blend that can be used as a tea or a tincture.

Rubella Formula

Mix together in a jar ½ ounce of each of the following herbs:

Nettles
Licorice
Calendula flowers
Cleavers
Spearmint

Add 1 tablespoon of the mix to 1 pint of boiling water, steep for 10 minutes, and strain. Mix with 4 ounces of apple juice. This may be taken warm or cool, several times a day.

- Herbal baths or washes made from infusions and decoctions will decrease any discomfort and itch. The following herbs are effective: burdock root, calendula flowers, comfrey root, lavender, or yarrow flowers.
- Herbal waters such as rose water, orange flower water, and distilled witch hazel can be dabbed on with cotton balls or added to a warm bath.

SCARLET FEVER

Some sore throats are caused by a certain type of bacteria called Group A beta-hemolytic streptococci. These bacteria produce a toxin that causes a rash typical of scarlet fever. The incubation period for scarlet fever is two to five days and is passed from child to child through oral and nasal secretions. It may be spread by a carrier who has no symptoms of the disease.

The onset is sudden, beginning with a headache, fever up to 104°F, sore throat, possible spots in the throat, swollen lymph nodes in the neck, abdominal pain, and vomiting. The rash develops in twenty-four to seventy-two hours, appearing as fine raised red spots, resembling course red sandpaper. It appears on the nape of the neck, in the armpits, and on the groin, then travels to the extremities. The rash lasts three to fourteen days.

Diagnosis requires a throat swab to confirm the bacteria type, but more often it is made simply on the appearance of the rash.

Treatments

To help resolve the infection, give immune-supporting herbs such as echinacea, usnea, astragalus, and garlic. For the fever combine with catnip, yarrow flowers, meadowsweet, linden flowers, or elder flowers. To improve lymphatic drainage and aid release of toxins from the skin, add cleavers, calendula, burdock, or peppermint. For irritability and restlessness, include skullcap, chamomile, lavender, or catnip.

Scarlet Fever Formula
2 parts echinacea tincture or glycerite
1 part garlic syrup
1 part peppermint tincture
1 part astragalus tincture or glycerite
1 part cleavers glycerite
1 part skullcap glycerite
½ part catnip tincture
½ part elder flowers tincture

Give ½ to 1 teaspoon, 4 times a day. This same formula can be made with dried herbs as an infusion and sweetened with honey. (See Making Herbal Preparations, starting on page 259.)

- Give immune-supporting vitamins and minerals in the following doses: vitamin C, 200 to 500 milligrams, 3 times a day; zinc, 10 to 15 milligrams, daily; and bioflavonoids, 100 to 500 milligrams, daily.
- Give lots of fluids; have the child sip water, diluted fruit juice, or herbal teas or punches, frequently. This keeps the throat moist and checks the fever. Avoid solid foods when the fever is high; give soups and juices instead.
- Herbal popsicles made from medicinal herbs and fruit juice are a great way to offer fluids and cool the discomfort in the throat and mouth. Use frozen teas made from chamomile, cleavers, elder flowers, spearmint, licorice, lemon balm, wintergreen, red clover, and linden flowers. Add fruit juice to sweeten.
- Use the Mullein/Lobelia Neck Wrap, 1 or 2 times a day. (See Recipes and Remedies for Infants and Children, starting on page 265.)
- Warm gargles made from infusions of myrrh, witch hazel, sage, rosemary, echinacea, and goldenseal can be used several times a day.

Bitter Orange Gargle
Combine in a 2-ounce amber bottle

½ oz. of calendula succus
½ oz. of peppermint tincture
¼ oz. of myrrh tincture
¼ oz. of goldenseal tincture
¼ oz. of cinnamon tincture
¼ oz. of bitter orange oil

Use ½ teaspoon of the bitter orange mix in 2 ounces of warm water. Gargle and swallow, 3 to 5 times a day.

SINUSITIS

Sinusitis can be either acute or chronic. Acute sinusitis is an inflammation or infection of the sinuses—the air-filled cavities in the face that connect the nasal passages. It is accompanied by one or several of the following symptoms: pain and swelling of the face, headache, stuffed nose, opaque to yellow-green nasal discharge, fever, and cough. With chronic or long-term sinusitis, fluid in the sinuses does not clear, the membranes swell, and there is constant nasal discharge or postnasal drip. Chronic sinusitis will often lead to an increase in acute sinus infections because the constant fluid and inflammation make one more susceptible to infection.

Because the sinuses are a continuation of the nasal cavity, they are affected by any infection of the nose or allergic reaction in the nose. Sometimes, a virus or an allergy attack that affects the sinus openings will induce a secondary bacterial infection. If a child gets frequent acute sinus infections with periods of constant nasal discharge in between, it is important to treat the sinuses for chronic sinusitis as well as to treat the acute episodes. By working to improve immune system health and resolve chronic inflammation in the nasal passages and possible allergies, the episodes of acute infection will occur less often.

Chronic sinusitis is often linked to food, dust, pet, or pollen allergies. This leads to chronic inflammation of the sinus and nasal mucous membranes and a reduced local immune response. The key is to eliminate food allergies or foods that are known to be irritating to the immune system, stabilize inflammation in the body, and build up the membranes and local immune response with diet, herbs, vitamins, and minerals. (See Part II, Working with the Young Immune System, starting on page 19.)

Treatments

- Give immune-supporting vitamins and minerals in the following doses: vitamin C, 200 to 500 milligrams, 3 times a day; zinc, 10 to 15 milligrams, daily; bioflavonoids, 100 to 500 milligrams, daily; and beta-carotene, 10,000 to 25,000 I.U., daily.
- During attacks of acute sinusitis, avoid dairy products—especially milk, cheese, and ice cream—as they increase mucous production in the body and make the body sluggish. Avoid other foods that are immune stressors like refined sugars, processed foods, citrus fruits, and refined wheat products. Give vegetable soups, lots of garlic and onions, and whole-grain porridges.
- Have the child drink a lot of fluids to encourage flushing of the kidneys and mucous membranes. Offer diluted fruit juices, herbal teas or punches, and abundant amounts of water. Choose herbs that support the immune response in fighting the infection such as astragalus, echinacea, garlic, and wild indigo. Mix with herbs that aid the local immune response in the sinuses like elder flowers, calendula, and chamomile. Add anti-inflammatory herbs like fenugreek seed and licorice and antiseptic herbs like garlic, goldenseal, rosemary, or thyme. Last, add a little ginger or cinnamon to the formula to increase circulation and warmth to the area.
- Use herbal inhalers or steams made from aromatic herbs high in essential oils like eucalyptus leaves, lavender flowers, rosemary, sage, thyme, or yarrow flowers. These essen-

tial oil plants will help to loosen mucus, stimulate a watery secretion from the membranes, and decrease microbial activity, helping to resolve the infection. Place a few drops of oil on a cotton ball and place at the entrance of a steam vaporizer to infuse the room where the child is sleeping.

- Apply hot packs to the face to relieve the discomfort, break up the congestion, and drain the sinuses. Use herbal compresses soaked in infusions of ginger, yarrow flowers, or eucalyptus to warm the area and white oak bark and witch hazel bark to dry the area. A sinus rub can be applied to the face over the sinus areas and covered with a hot cloth or hot water bottle. Castor oil packs also work well.

- Elder/Eyebright Formula (available from Gaia Herbs) is a combination of elder flowers and berries to give all the benefits from both medicinally active parts of the elder shrub. These are mixed with decongesting herbs and mucous membrane tonics, eyebright, fenugreek, and plantain. Thyme and aniseed are added for their warming antimicrobial and antiseptic properties. I find the formula to be effective in all types of sinusitis including viral, bacterial, allergic, or inflammatory. Doses by age are on the bottle.

Herbal Sinus Rub

Mix in a 2-ounce amber bottle:

½ oz. St. John's wort oil
1 Tbs. lobelia oil
1 Tbs. bayberry root tincture
1 Tbs. myrrh tincture
1 Tbs. goldenseal tincture
1 tsp. cayenne oil or tincture

Shake well before use. Apply topically, with heat, 1 to 3 times a day.

SLEEPLESSNESS/INSOMNIA

Generally, a child requires more sleep than an adult, an average of ten to twelve hours per night. However, the younger the child, the more likely it is that he or she will awaken in the night for feeding or comfort.

There are many different causes for sleep disturbances that should be investigated if your child is having problems sleeping. For example, children with food or airborne allergies often have trouble breathing during sleep, which wakes them. They also may have trouble falling asleep, or they may awaken because of a bad dream, stomachache, or frequent urination.

The hyperactive child often has a hard time falling asleep and often only sleeps a few hours. The emotionally upset or worried child may be bothered by nightmares or fear of the dark or being alone and may need a parent to sleep with him or her until the crisis passes. Acute infections, such as earache, sinusitis, or fevers, can cause restlessness and fitful sleep. Chronic skin rashes, asthma, or nasal congestion will also disturb a child's sleep patterns.

Treatments

When treating sleep disturbances, it is important to figure out what is producing the symptom of sleeplessness. Finding the cause and treating it will ultimately lead to a regular sleep cycle. At the same time, the use of herbal treatments to induce sleep and relaxation can be helpful.

- Avoid foods that act to stimulate such as chocolate, caffeinated drinks, sugar, food additives and colorings, and processed foods. Give a whole-food diet with lots of fresh vegetables to provide minerals. Calcium, magnesium, and zinc are particularly helpful.

- There are many lovely ways to use herbs to induce sleep. A warm tea given in the evening can relax and calm the child before bedtime. Many of the herbs that can be used in relaxing and calming teas or tinctures can also be used as a bedtime bath or mixed into a sleep pillow, where the pleasant scents of the herbs affect the nervous system. Choose herbs like catnip, chamomile, hops, lavender flowers, lemon balm, linden flowers, oats, passionflower, and skullcap for their calming effect on the nervous system and their relaxing effect on the body.

- Essential oils used in massage oils, baths, and infused into the air can have a strong effect on the nervous system as they find direct entry into the pleasure centers of the brain through the nose. Rubbing them on the body through massage gives the added benefit of relaxation to the body muscles and tissue and allows the child to be touched, which is comforting and calming. Add a few drops to a warm bath or make a bath oil by mixing it with sweet almond oil. (See Recipes and Remedies for Infants and Children, starting on page 265.) Try putting a few drops of oil on a lightbulb in the child's room. The warmth of the light will diffuse the oil and scent the room. Dropping a few drops into a pot of boiling water will also work. Choose oils such as chamomile, lavender, neroli, rose, sandlewood, or ylang-ylang.

Herbal Sleep and Dream Pillows

Mix together ½ cup each of lavender flowers, linden flowers, and rosebuds. Add ¼ cup each of hops, mugwort, and sweet woodruff. Fill small pillows made out of a soft, pretty cloth with the herb mix. Place the pillows close to the sleeping child's head.

Herbal Tea for Sleep
Mix together the following ingredients:
1 part aniseed
1 part chamomile flowers
1 part linden flowers
½ part hops
½ part passionflower

Use 1 teaspoon per cup of boiling water. Let steep 10 minutes, strain, and serve. Sweeten with fruit juice, if necessary.

SORE THROAT AND TONSILLITIS

A sore throat may be caused by any type of infection that affects the upper respiratory system, which includes the nose, sinuses, ears, and lungs. Most sore throats are caused by viral infections and less frequently by bacterial infections. The most common bacteria to infect the throat is streptococcus. These can be seen in a throat culture. If your child has a fever, a very sore red throat, and swollen glands, see your doctor. Viral throat infections are often accompanied by runny eyes and nose and a cough.

Allergies to airborne substances like dust, pollen, and dander as well as food allergies can cause a sore throat. Often the throat is sore upon waking or at the end of the day. In the winter season, the heating system can dry the air out and cause a morning sore throat that goes away after being up a few hours. Humidifying the air can help to eliminate this.

A sore throat is also the presenting complaint of a child with tonsillitis. Tonsillitis is a swelling and infection of the tonsils and adenoids. This may be acute or chronic. The tonsils and adenoids are part of the lymphatic system and are found at the entrance of the throat at the back of the mouth. They fight against infection and pollution entering the body through the mouth and nasal passages. In acute tonsillitis, the tonsils become inflamed, tender, and suddenly swollen; the back of the throat becomes sore; the neck lymph glands swell; and there is general malaise. Tonsillitis may accompany a cold, influenza virus, or a bacterial upper respiratory infection. Chronic tonsillitis occurs when the tonsils stay constantly enlarged and there are frequent bouts of acute tonsillitis. Chronic tonsillitis is often associated with allergies. When the tonsils remain enlarged, it is a sign that the glands are working all the time and have a backup of waste stored in the gland. The more frequently the child is exposed to the allergen, the more likely the tonsils will become enlarged. The best approach to chronic tonsillitis is to build up the immune system; support the lymphatic system with herbs like calendula flowers, burdock root, and cleavers; and address the allergy or food intolerance.

Treatments

- Give immune-supporting vitamins and minerals in the following doses: vitamin C, 200 to 500 milligrams, 3 times a day; zinc, 10 to 15 milligrams, daily; bioflavonoids, 100 to 500 milligrams, daily; and beta-carotene, 10,000 to 25,000 I.U., daily.
- Herbal treatment of a sore throat should aim to support the immune system in fighting the infection and the lymphatic system in draining and defending the area as well as relieving the discomfort. Herbal teas, tinctures, syrups, and glycerites are useful preparations for this. Immune and antiseptic herbs include astragalus root, echinacea root, garlic, goldenseal root, licorice root, thyme, and wild indigo. Mix them with lymphatic herbs like burdock, calendula,

cleavers, and nettles and analgesic herbs like wintergreen, willow, cayenne pepper, cloves, or meadowsweet.

- Slippery elm or zinc lozenges can be sucked on frequently throughout the day.
- Warm infusions of rosemary, sage, and thyme can be used as an antiseptic gargle. Add a dash of cayenne pepper or ginger powder. Gargle 3 or 4 times a day.
- Throat Spray (available from Gaia's Children) is a mix of herbs that can be sprayed directly on the back of the throat through a pump nozzle, making it very easy to use. My four-year-old niece, Mia, thinks this is the "best medicine" I've come up with yet. Finding the pump nozzle particularly appealing, it gives small children a chance to "do it themselves," which can also be appealing to that age.
- Rub warming Vaporous Rub (available from Gaia Herbs) on the skin of the front and sides of the throat and behind the ears to stimulate the lymph system to drain and provide some relief from the discomfort of swollen glands.

Immune and Lymphatic Syrup for Sore Throats
½ oz. echinacea tincture
½ oz. garlic syrup
½ oz. licorice tincture
½ oz. thyme glycerite
½ oz. cleavers glycerite
1 Tbs. calendula succus
1 Tbs. wintergreen tincture

Mix well and store in an amber-colored glass bottle. Give ½ to 1 teaspoon, 4 times a day. This same formula can be made as an infusion and sweetened with honey.

Calendula/Bitter Orange Gargle or Throat Paint
Bitter orange oil is highly antiseptic, reducing bacterial and viral infection. This makes an excellent mixture to paint on

the throat with cotton swabs a few times a day. I recommend it for viral and bacterial throat infection, including strep throat. Mix in a 1-ounce bottle the following ingredients.

½ oz. calendula succus
1 Tbs. echinacea tincture
1 tsp. goldenseal tincture or glycerite
1 tsp. bitter orange oil

Shake well before using, as the oil will float to the top of the bottle. Use 30 to 60 drops in 2 ounces of warm water, gargle, and swallow.

Mullein/Lobelia Neck Wrap for Sore Throats, Tonsillitis, and Laryngitis

1 oz. verbascum leaf
½ oz. lobelia
1 tsp. cayenne
1 pint apple cider vinegar
1 pint water

Put vinegar, water, mullein, and lobelia into a pot, cover, and simmer gently for 15 minutes; turn off the heat and add the cayenne. Dip a cloth into the mixture and wrap the neck. Cover the wrap with plastic and then a dry towel to keep the heat in. Dip the cloth again in the warm liquid when cool. Use 1 to 2 times daily, for 10 to 15 minutes each application.

Carrot Poultice for Sore Throats

Grate 2 large carrots. Spread onto a thin cloth (such as cheesecloth) and fold the cloth so that the carrot is enclosed. Wrap around throat and secure with safety pin. Cover with an additional scarf or towel. Poultice can be either hot or cold, depending on which feels better.

For cold, combine crushed ice with the carrot.

For hot, place cloth and carrot in hot water and squeeze out before applying to neck.

SPRAINS

A sprain is a partial or complete tear of a ligament marked by pain, swelling, bruising, decreased joint motion, and mild internal bleeding. Sprains are common during childhood, often occurring in the wrists, ankles, fingers, toes, neck, and back. Consult your doctor for serious sprains.

Treatments

- Ice and elevation are effective first-aid measures for the first twenty-four hours. It is important to immobilize the injured part and avoid using it for several days.
- Apply arnica cream or oil to the area several times a day.

Liniment for Sprains
½ oz. lobelia oil
½ oz. St. John's wort oil
½ oz. wormwood oil
1 Tbs. ginger oil
1 Tbs. cayenne oil

Apply over area, 3 times a day, with a light massage.

STOMACHACHES

Childhood stomachaches seem to be a normal part of growing up. Most children complain of a tummyache at least once in their lives. Stomachaches can be divided into two categories: acute stomachache of sudden onset or chronic ongoing stomachache, which is often intermittent. Both acute and chronic stomachaches can have many causes, including eating the wrong foods, overeating, digestive infection, constipation, diarrhea, colic, food allergies, food poisoning, motion sickness, overexcitement, anxiety, nervousness, prolonged hiccups, muscle strain, urinary tract infection, appendicitis, hepatitis, and meningitis.

If your child is complaining of acute stomach pain, it is important to determine the source of the pain if possible. Try asking the following questions:

1. Has your child had a recent bowel movement, and if so, was it hard or loose? If this is the case, treat for constipation (see page 100) or diarrhea (see page 114).
2. Has your child been exposed to anyone with similar symptoms, or have the children at school had similar symptoms? If so, treat for infection.
3. Has your child eaten any foods that may have been soiled or contaminated with a food-poisoning bacteria? If so, treat for food poisoning.
4. Has your child had a recent upset or stressful experience? If so, treat with relaxants and nervines.
5. Does your child have any urinary complaints or symptoms? If so, treat for urinary tract infection (see page 190).
6. Does your child display any other types of symptoms or cannot explain the source of the pain? If so, see your health care provider.

Chronic stomachaches are most often due to food intolerances, constipation, or emotional stress. Some chronic stomachaches can be caused by digestive inflammatory disease, lead poisoning, worm infestation, and low-grade infections. Often, emotional stress causes abdominal pain around the belly button area and is accompanied by no other symptoms. Stressful or anxiety-producing situations for children come in a variety of shapes and colors, so take a moment to really look at what the situation may be. It could be a holiday, a new baby, school, an upset with a friend, the selling of a home, anticipation of an event, a family argument, or an emotion such as sorrow or anger.

Treatments

- Avoid giving solid foods until the pain is gone. Give vegetable broths and warm herbal teas or punches made from aniseed, cardamon seed, cinnamon, cloves, ginger, and meadowsweet.
- Use digestive relaxants like chamomile, catnip, hops, lemon balm, linden flowers, or wintergreen to relieve abdominal tension when the upset is due to emotional stress or anxiety.
- If digestive infection is from bacteria or virus, use syrups, teas, or tinctures of antimicrobial herbs like echinacea, garlic, hyssop, licorice, sage, or thyme. Give a dose every 2 hours.
- Apply heat to the stomach with a warm compress soaked in crampbark and lavender; use a hot water bottle or a heating pad. Castor oil packs can be very comforting or rub the stomach gently with a warm aromatic massage oil.
- One of my favorite formulas for upset stomach, gas, spasms, nausea, or indigestion is a combination of chamomile flowers, lemon balm herb, spearmint leaves, catnip herb, fennel seed, and gingerroot (Gaia Children makes a formula with these ingredients called Tummy Tonic). I give it diluted in water and have the child sip it slowly.
- Several homeopathic remedies can be used, depending on the symptoms. Carbo vegetabilis can be used for the child who has gas, burping, stomach distention, pain in the cen-

ter of the abdomen, and indigestion. Give 3 pellets per dose of 6c or 12c, and repeat in a half hour if necessary. Nux vomica may be used for the child who has eaten too many sweets or has otherwise overindulged. The child is often irritable, with a headache and often a congested bowel. Arsenicum alba can be used for treating signs of food poisoning or stomachache accompanied by diarrhea. Both of these remedies can be used in a 6c or 12c strength, given in a dose of 3 pellets, and repeated in a half hour to an hour if needed.

- Proflora such as lactobacillus acidophilus can help restore normal healthy intestinal flora. It can be used to treat an acute stomachache as well as chronic complaints and should be used for several weeks after digestive infection or food poisoning.

STRESS

Ideally, we would like to think of childhood as being a time of little stress, carefree days, and laughter. We all know this is far from the truth, and children have their share of stress. Stressors, or things that can trigger a stress response in the body, can come in many shapes and forms. There are what I refer to as natural stressors such as cold weather, heat, lack of food, and infections. These to some degree affect everyone. Yet if one chooses, they can lessen the effects of these stressors by wearing the right clothing, not skipping meals, and so forth. Another type of stressor may be found in the environment in the forms of heavy metals, pesticides, chemicals, smoke, hormones, and so on. Then there are those stressors that come with lifestyle, such as moving, peers, school, sports, family, physical trauma, emotional trauma, or allergies. The effects of stress can be long term or short term, and the more the body is exposed to long-term stress, the more adapting the body must do to cope with the needs it has during this time. It can become a vicious cycle.

Physical symptoms of stress can impact almost any system in the body, and most often several systems are affected at once. Here are some of the more common ways stress can express itself in children:

- Anger, irritability, mood swings, emotional outbursts
- Apathy
- Anxiety, depression
- Addictive behaviors
- Bed-wetting
- Back pain, stomach pain, muscle pain
- Lack of appetite, overeating, nausea or upset stomach, bowel changes
- Headache, neck pain, migraine
- Insomnia, restlessness, oversleeping
- Inability to concentrate, forgetfulness
- Fatigue, burned-out feeling
- Feeling overwhelmed or helpless
- Pounding heart; rapid pulse; rapid, shallow breathing
- Skin rash
- Teeth grinding
- Tightness in chest or belly

As you can see from the list, many of these symptoms can also have other causes, and identifying the source is important. Talk to your child.

Physiologically, the adrenal gland is an important player in the regulation of stress in the body. If a person undergoes long-term stress, the gland can become less and less able to deal with the effects in a healthy way, and the body beings to show signs of not coping. Many of the communication lines start to fail in the nervous system, immune system, and endocrine system, thus weakening the body's other defense mechanisms. That's one of the reasons why people can experience physical symptoms from long-term stress after the stressful situation has resolved, as in post-traumatic stress syndrome.

Treatments

Because stress can come in so many forms and fashions, treatments for dealing with stress must come in a variety as well. The goals should include lessening stressful situations if possible, including stress-relieving activities, making good lifestyle choices, and physical exercise. For specific treatments for specific symptoms, see that complaint.

Lifestyle Recommendations

- Regular exercise on a daily basis or martial arts can be very helpful, as is getting outside in the air and sunlight. Swimming is a good form of exercise, along with having the added value of the calming effects of the water.
- Laughter is a wonderful medicine and finding something fun and humorous can have a beneficial effect on one's mood. Try to engage your child daily in some good old-fashioned laughter.
- Be sure your child is breathing full and completely; often, we tend to swallow breath or breathe from the top of our lungs. Teach your child how to breathe deeply into the base of the lungs, feeling the belly push outward with each deep breath.
- Encourage a regular bedtime to ensure sufficient rest. Use relaxing herbs like chamomile, catnip, hops, skullcap, lemon balm, lavender, or valerian as teas or extracts to

encourage sleep. Try Gaia's Children Passionflower/Lemon Balm Formula for a premixed, over-the-counter product.

Dietary Recommendations

- One factor that can stimulate an internal stress response is when the blood sugar drops too low. This can happen to many children who overeat simple carbohydrates, have low-protein diets, or go too long without eating. So, eating three regular meals, not skipping meals (especially breakfast), and eating a good whole-food diet with adequate protein are recommended.
- Avoid soda pop, sugary foods and simple carbohydrates, caffeine, artificial colors and preservatives, and overeating.
- Eat whole-grain oats in the form of cereals and breads. Oatmeal with sliced nuts and maple sugar is a great breakfast. Oats are great for the nervous system and act to stabilize the blood sugar.
- If you think your child suffers from a hypoglycemic drop during the day or night, see a nutritionist to get some hints on foods and eating schedules. Often, the best management strategies for hypoglycemic episodes include regular food intake, good protein levels, complex carbohydrates, and limited simple carbohydrates.

Supplementation

Stress can take a toll on the cells, tissues, organs, and systems of the body. The adrenal gland plays a key role in coping with stress and can suffer as a result of high levels of stress. Vitamin B complex, vitamin C, essential fatty acids, potassium, magnesium, and zinc are all important nutrients for adrenal health. Supplementation of these during long-term stress or high-stress times would be recommended. (See Essential Nutrients, page 39.)

Herbal Treatments

- Adaptogen herbs are highly recommended as part of any plan to counteract the effects of stress. Two herbs that come to mind are Siberian ginseng and ashwagandha; they can be used alone or mixed together.
- Herbs that support adrenal function such as licorice root, Siberian ginseng, nettle leaf, and rosehips will act to improve glandular function during times of wear and tear.
- Tonic herbs that act to strengthen and enhance vitality, support the body's elimination channels, improve circulation, and balance function of the systems should also be included in the treatment plan. Think of plants like nettles, red clover blossoms, astragalus root, and oats.
- Nervine herbs can be useful during times of stress or to deal with some of the symptoms such as insomnia, headache, restlessness, or nervousness. Herbs that act as a nervine, calming and relaxing the nerves, muscles, and mind, can also have a rejuvenating or tonic affect. I recommend lavender flowers, skullcap, oats, linden flowers, and lemon balm.

Chronic Stress Formula

This formula is designed to support and rebalance the body's own mechanisms for stress management, including the nervous system, adrenal gland, and immune system. Use it with chronic illness, post-trauma, during periods of convalescence after surgery, when taking antibiotics, or when experiencing severe acute illness. Give ¼ to ½ teaspoon of the formula in warm water or spearmint tea. Use 1 to 3 times a day, for several weeks to 2 months.

Mix together the following herbal extracts:

½ oz. ashwagandha tincture
½ oz. astragalus tincture
½ oz. Siberian ginseng tincture
½ oz. oat (*Avena sativa*) glycerite
½ oz. skullcap glycerite
¼ oz. licorice root tincture
¼ oz. nettle glycerite
¼ oz. lavender flowers glycerite

STYES

Styes are localized infections in the follicle of an eyelash or a gland in the eyelid. There is localized redness and swelling, producing a small pustule, with discomfort or itching. The infection is often bacterial in origin, and several may occur at one time. They may spread through contact from person to person. Wash your hands after applying topical treatment to the sty.

Treatments

- Apply localized heat to the area by using compresses soaked in soothing, astringent, antiseptic herbs to help resolve the infection and heal the sore. Apply the hot herbal compresses 3 or 4 times a day, for 20 minutes. Cotton balls soaked in the herbs covered with a warm washcloth work well. Choose 1 or 2 from the following list and make an infusion to soak the compresses in:

Calendula flowers

Eyebright herb

Goldenseal root

Myrrh resin

Witch hazel leaf or bark

Yarrow flowers

- A paste made from powdered slippery elm, goldenseal, and bentonite mixed with enough water to make it creamy can be applied to the sty, 1 or 2 times a day.

SUNBURN

Sunburn is a thermal burn from exposure to the radiation of the sun. It is usually a first-degree burn involving the outer layer of the skin, the epidermis. Radiation from the sun comes in two forms of ultraviolet rays: UVA and UVB. Both are damaging to the skin, even though UVB rays are most present during the summer. Precautions to prevent sunburn should be used all year-round. Overexposure to the sun will produce red, hot, painful skin. If blisters appear, then the burn has reached the deeper layers of the skin. Sun poisoning may occur from overexposure to the sun, causing a hivelike rash over the burn, fever, nausea, and malaise. Call your doctor immediately for treatment.

The best treatment for sunburn is prevention; this means taking precautions before going into the sun. Do not overexpose the skin. Put a hat on your child to protect the face, put a light T-shirt on your child if she has sensitive skin, and use a natural sunscreen with an SPF of 10 or higher. Apply the sunscreen every several hours when out all day and after swimming to give full protection during exposure. Remember, cloudy or hazy days will still allow the ultraviolet rays to come through.

Treatments

- Soak in a cool bath as soon as possible after sun exposure. Add strong herbal infusions made from cooling, soothing herbs such as strawberry leaves, comfrey root or leaves, and marshmallow root.
- Apply a compress soaked in mucilage of comfrey root for 20 minutes, several times a day. (See recipe, page 266.)
- Apply 100-percent aloe vera gel or fresh mucilage from a leaf of a living plant. Cut the leaf the long way to expose more of the gel. Apply several times a day.
- Oatmeal bath or Aveeno (available at your local pharmacy) can be very soothing and cooling to the skin. Use ½ to 1 cup of oatmeal in a clean cotton sock, drop into the bath, and squeeze a few times to release the oatmeal juice into the bath water.
- Use cocoa butter and coconut oil–based lotions and creams to moisten, soften, and replenish nutrients to the skin after exposure. Make your own after-the-sun lotion or cream by gently heating the oil or cocoa butter in a double boiler and adding fresh comfrey leaves, plantain leaves, and calendula flowers. Keep on very low heat for 20 to 30 minutes, and strain through gauze while warm. Mix in some aloe gel as it cools before it is too firm. Store in the refrigerator during the summer.
- Herbal oils made from diffusing fresh or dry herbs in olive oil with a little vitamin E oil added works great. Try St. John's wort, chamomile flowers, and yarrow flowers to help heal the burned skin and stimulate new skin growth.

- Give homeopathic cantharis 6c or 12c, 3 pellets, 3 times a day. This will reduce the intensity of the burn and prevent the uncomfortable symptoms.
- Give vitamin C with bioflavonoids and omega 3 oil supplementation, 2 times a day, for several weeks after sunburn. This will help to encourage normal skin growth and boost the immune system.

TEETHING

Babies usually start teething at five to six months old. A baby usually will cut twenty teeth during the first three years of life. These teeth are temporary and are partly formed within the gums at birth. The age and sequence of the eruption of teeth vary greatly from child to child, but often the lower incisors are the first to break through. The upper four incisors and the lower lateral incisors usually follow. Next come the one-year molars, the canines, and then the two-year molars.

Teething commonly is accompanied by symptoms of dribbling, chewing on fingers and objects, red swollen gums, fretfulness, irritability, clinginess, sleep disturbances, facial rash, lack of appetite, and bowel changes. The increase in saliva, gum inflammation, or other symptoms may predispose the child to secondary illness or symptoms of fever, earache, upper respiratory infection, yellowish nasal discharge, diarrhea, or cough. If your child is teething and has these accompanying symptoms, be sure that the teething symptoms are not masking an illness.

Treatments

- Give herbs to reduce discomfort, soothe inflammation, and support the immune system. This helps to avoid secondary infection and fever. Use calendula flowers, catnip, echinacea, elder flowers, meadowsweet, lemon balm, or usnea. Mix these with herbs such as chamomile flowers, linden flowers, willow bark, or wintergreen leaves to calm and decrease the pain. These herbs can be used as teas, popsicles, glycerites, or tinctures. Freezing the tea in ice cube trays or popsicles, or saturating a washcloth with an herbal blend and freezing it are great ways to apply the herb to the gums. The cold also is beneficial as an anti-inflammatory and pain reliever.

- Herbal chewing sticks are long thin pieces of licorice root or marshmallow root that can be given to the baby to chew on. The sweet taste of both the herbs is very pleasant.
- Try teething tablets. Several combination homeopathic remedies for teething are available in health food stores and can be given to help relieve the symptoms of teething. Give tablets or drops, 4 times a day or at bedtime.
- Make an herbal gum rub. The gums can be rubbed with a dab of honey combined with a drop of essential oil of clove or wintergreen. This will help to numb the gums and reduce the swelling. Gums may be rubbed 2 to 3 times a day.
- Gummy Rub (available from Gaia's Children) is a topical gum rub that has a thick consistency, which makes it easy to apply to the gums without running off. This rub has analgesic, anti-inflammatory, and numbing effects on the local gum area. I have also found this rub to be useful for older children after having their braces adjusted. Apply with a cotton swab, several times a day and before bed.

THRUSH

Thrush is a fungal infection of the mouth caused by a yeast-like fungus, *Candida albicans*. This fungus can also cause diaper rash; red irritated skin in the folds of baby's neck, thighs, and underarms; and vaginal yeast infection. Thrush is most common with infants younger than six months and is usually associated with immune-deficiency states in older children and adults. Thrush, if severe, can lead to breast-feeding troubles, so it is best to treat and resolve it as soon as possible.

Thrush presents as white, curdlike patches on the tongue, insides of the cheeks, gums, and lips that do not wipe away. If the patch is scraped away it leaves a red, irritated sore that may bleed. Avoid scraping the patches; this will make matters worse. This condition can be painful and cause the child to lose his appetite or refuse to nurse well. If the baby is nursing, the nipple of the breast could also be infected with candida, and that can set up a vicious cycle of reinfection for mother and baby. It is most important to treat the baby and the mother and to practice good hygiene, washing the nipple before and after each feeding and always remembering to dry the nipple well. Air the nipples daily to aid in diminishing the yeast growth. If the baby uses a bottle or pacifier, then these must also be cleaned regularly. Washing in a dishwasher or cleaning with hydrogen peroxide followed by a water rinse works well.

Thrush is often seen after antibiotic use by the baby or a breast-feeding mother. The antibiotics disrupt the normal flora in the baby's mouth and digestive system, allowing the yeast to grow more easily. (See Antibiotics and the Immune System, page 27.) Using profloras, like lactobacillus acidophilus, while on antibiotics can help keep the yeast from overgrowing. Breast-feeding mothers who are dealing with thrush or a yeast infection of the nipples should also supplement their diet with proflora along with eating live-culture plain, unsweetened yogurt daily.

Treatments

- Irrigate the infant's mouth with a mixture of water and lactobacillus bifidus several times a day. Use 1 capsule to 4 ounces of warm water, and use the whole amount over the course of a day. Repeat daily until all patches are gone. Use a needleless syringe or an eyedropper to put it into baby's mouth.

- Swab the inside of the child's mouth with the following mixture: 5 drops each of black walnut tincture, blood root tincture, and spilanthes tincture in 1 ounce of warm water. Swab the mouth several times a day, followed by a lacto-bacillus rinse. This may also be used to wipe the nipples with after feeding as well.

- Gentain violet in a 1-percent solution can be used for persistent cases to swab out the baby's mouth or to apply to the nipple. Gentain violet stains, so use with care.

- Breast-feeding mothers should consider a low-sugar, low-yeast, and low-carbohydrate diet, avoiding such things as breads, sweets, baked goods, concentrated fruit juices, soda and pasta, and focus on whole grains, fresh vegetables, and good protein sources for a few weeks while treating candida.

URINARY TRACT INFECTIONS

Infections of the urinary tract are common during childhood. They occur more frequently in girls than in boys due to the difference in the urethra length. About 5 percent of girls get urinary tract infections before the age of maturity. Urinary tract infections in babies may be caused by a structural abnormality somewhere along the urinary tract. This may cause a partial or total block in the flow of urine, resulting in the reflux of stagnant urine from the bladder leaking back into the kidney. Most often, urinary tract infections are caused by the bacteria *E. coli*, which is found normally in large amounts in the bowel. The bacteria may travel along the perineal area from the rectal area to the urethral opening. Improper wiping, diapers, constipation, and touching are all ways of spreading the bacteria. Some urinary tract infections may be caused by yeast from the vaginal area. The infection can affect the urethra, the bladder (cystitis), or the kidney.

A urinary tract infection may elicit no symptoms at all. This is known as a silent UTI. Common symptoms associated with urinary tract infection include any one or combination of the following: urgency, frequency or pain with urination, dribbling of urine, bed-wetting, daytime incontinence, foul-smelling urine, cloudy or bloody urine, fever, low-back pain, abdominal pain, vomiting, or malaise.

Urinary tract infections may be low grade and hard to diagnose if symptoms are vague. The doctor can run a urinalysis to identify the infectious agent for an accurate diagnosis. If left untreated, it may occur again after a few weeks. If your child does not respond to treatments after a few days or the symptoms worsen, fever is persistent, or low-back pain presents, see your doctor. Chronic urinary tract infection can be a symptom of food allergy or candida overgrowth.

Treatments

- Make sure to have the child drink lots of water and herbal teas. Avoid fruit juice due to the high sugar content. Unsweetened cranberry juice can be helpful in keeping the infection from spreading up the urinary tract. The cranberry helps to make the tract slippery so that the bacteria cannot hold on. Use 2 to 4 ounces, 2 times a day. Have your child drink at least 1 cup of water or herbal tea each hour. Adding lemon to the water can be helpful.
- Using herbal medicines that are diuretic will help to stimulate the flow of urine and flush out the system. Common diuretic herbs include uva ursi, couch grass, cornsilk, dandelion leaf, parsley, horsetail, and nettles. Horsetail, uva

ursi, and nettles are also astringent in their action and will help to soothe any inflammation.

- Herbs that are soothing in quality, such as marshmallow root, cornsilk, slippery elm, and couch grass, will be especially useful in reducing inflammation, irritability, and hot or burning pain. I prefer to give these separately in their own tea or tincture. Otherwise, the tea or tincture may get stringy or lumpy due to the mixture of plant constituents.
- Combine antiseptic herbs to fight the infection. The aromatic herbs containing essential oils work well as urinary antiseptics because as the body excretes them into the urine they naturally carry their antiseptic and antimicrobial action to the infected area. Some of the herbs I like to use include thyme, hyssop, rosemary, juniper berry, and yarrow.
- Give immune-supporting vitamins and minerals in the following doses: vitamin C, 200 to 500 milligrams, 3 times a day; zinc, 10 to 15 milligrams, daily; and bioflavonoids, 100 to 500 milligrams, daily.

Marshmallow Syrup

2 oz. marshmallow root, sliced
½–1 cup sugar
1 cup distilled water

Soak marshmallow root in water for 12 hours. Add sugar and heat to a boil, cool, and strain through a cheesecloth. Bottle and store in the refrigerator. Use ½ to 1 teaspoon, 4 times a day.

Barley Water

Useful for soothing urinary irritation and increasing urination. Soak ½ pound of barley in 1 quart water for 12 hours or simmer until soft. Strain. Sweeten with honey if desired. Give several cups of barley water a day.

VOMITING

Vomiting is a common occurrence during childhood. It is a symptom that on its own is usually not a problem unless it leads to dehydration. Vomiting does not usually cause dehydration in an otherwise healthy child unless there is associated copious diarrhea for a duration of forty-eight hours or longer. Determining the reason for the vomiting is important in the overall treatment of the illness.

Commonly, infants regurgitate or vomit when overfed. This is normally not a problem if weight gain is good and it diminishes as the infant matures. Excessive vomiting can be a sign of food intolerance to milk or formula and, if frequent and forceful, may be a sign of structural abnormality in the digestive tract. Infants may also vomit due to gas in the stomach, weak stomach, or infection.

Toddlers may vomit because of food intolerance, overeating, allergic reaction, overexcitement, food poisoning, viral infection, or infectious disease.

Colds and coughs with a lot of mucus or phlegm may cause vomiting due to the phlegm getting into the stomach or from a spastic cough trying to loosen or bring up phlegm from the lungs. In this case the vomit is mixed with mucus and watery secretions.

Vomiting caused by an infection usually comes on suddenly and is accompanied by fever. If due to overexcitement or overeating, the food is often undigested, and the stomach feels better once it has been emptied. Children with weak stomachs often vomit a little bit after feedings or frequently complain of an upset stomach. These children will benefit from supplementation of lactobacillus acidophilus and bifidus for several months and digestive-strengthening herbs like aniseed, cinnamon, gingerroot, fennel seed, peppermint, or spearmint, given regularly.

Treatments

- When your child is vomiting do not give solid foods or milk, as they will only make things worse. Encourage small sips or teaspoonfuls of cool, clear fluids, such as water, herbal teas, ginger ale, diluted fruit juices, or electrolyte drinks like Recharge. If a teaspoon of fluid is retained every 5 minutes, then the child will keep down 2 ounces of fluid over an hour. Start slowly to avoid overloading the stomach. Use clear liquids until vomiting stops for a period of 6 hours. Start feeding with a bland diet and vegetable broths. Avoid milk or milk products.
- Slippery elm given as a weak tea in teaspoon doses every 5 to 10 minutes or as a lozenge is often my first choice.
- There are many useful herbal medicines that will help to relieve nausea and vomiting and warm the stomach. Warm teas of any of the following or a combination of 2 or 3 will work nicely. Choose from aniseed, chamomile flowers, cinnamon, cloves, fennel seed, ginger, lemon balm, peppermint, raspberry leaf, or spearmint. These same herbs may be used in tincture or glycerite form by adding 5 to 10 drops to a little water and sipping it slowly.
- Applying a warm castor oil pack over the stomach for 30 minutes can soothe and decrease the stomach discomfort.

Anise/Ginger Drops
Mix 2 parts aniseed tincture to 1 part gingerroot tincture. Use 5 to 10 drops in a little water; sip every 10 minutes or so.

WARTS

Warts are solid, raised growths on the skin that are usually painless and range in size from one-quarter to one-half inch. They may grow anywhere on the body but mainly occur on the hands, feet, and face. Warts are usually caused by a virus and may be spread by contact, itching, and scratching. Most warts resolve on their own over a period of two to three years.

Treatments

- Topical applications are the most common route of treatment. Support the body's immune system with good nutrition, antioxidant vitamins and minerals, and using antiviral herbs like lemon balm, licorice, St. John's wort, or thuja.
- Apply a patch over the wart cut from a fresh banana peel, with the inner peel next to the skin; cover it with a Band-Aid and leave on overnight. Repeat for 3 nights. On the fourth night put a few drops of one of either liquid beta-carotene, tea tree oil, or a mixture of equal parts of witch hazel tincture, greater celandine tincture, and thuja tincture on the wart before applying the banana peel. Continue for 2 to 3 weeks. The wart should start to turn black as it begins to die.

WHOOPING COUGH

Whooping cough, or pertussis, is an acute, highly communicable bacterial disease characterized by a rapid series of spasmodic coughing fits that usually end in a prolonged, high-pitched, crowing inspiration (the whoop). Transmission is by aspiration of bacteria sprayed into the air by someone infected with the disease. The incubation period is usually seven to fourteen days but may be as long as twenty-one days.

The illness begins with a runny nose, low-grade fever, and an irritating nocturnal cough that builds in intensity over the next two to three weeks. Upper respiratory inflammation is characterized by increased mucous secretion. The second phase, the "paroxysmal stage," occurs when the characteristic whoop develops at the end of the cough. A common pattern might be five to fifteen rapidly consecutive spasmodic coughs followed by a whoop. These coughing bouts can last a minute or two and may cause vomiting or gagging of mucus, and the face may turn red or purple. One bout may follow another; activity and temperature changes can bring on coughing bouts. The illness has a six to eight week duration, which is divided into three stages:

1. Catarrhal stage: ten to fourteen days
2. Paroxysmal stage: until the fourth week
3. Convalescent stage: ends at about the eighth week

Whooping cough usually resolves spontaneously but is more serious in children under the age of two and in the elderly. As a child gets older and has a stronger immune system, the disease is usually less serious and severe.

Treatments

- The child should eat as little as possible. Overfeeding prolongs the disease. Small meals are best. In fact, a full fruit and vegetable juice fast, including clear vegetable broths, can be most helpful. Flavor a vegetable broth with fresh garlic and ginger and emphasize therapeutic foods such as garlic, onions, leeks, turnips, grapes, pineapples, and green leafy vegetables. Avoid cow's milk and other dairy products, white bread, refined or processed foods, sugar and sweets, and mucous-forming foods such as tofu, meat, ice cream, shellfish, fats, and vinegars.
- Give immune-supporting vitamins and minerals in the following doses: vitamin C, 200 to 500 milligrams, 3 times a

day; zinc, 10 to 15 milligrams, daily; and bioflavonoids, 100 to 500 milligrams, daily.

- Herbal treatments used for whooping cough feature a variety of preparations including teas, cough syrups, steams, chest rubs, and compresses. It is important to use several types of remedies regularly throughout the illness. If the illness is addressed in the first stage and responds well, the second stage, with the coughing episodes, will be less severe. If the cough is severe, then it is most important to apply the herbal medicines regularly and frequently throughout the day. In other words, the parent needs to be prepared to nurse the child full-time.

When the symptoms of a cold first appear in the infant or child use immune-supporting herbs such as astragalus, echinacea, garlic, linden flowers, and usnea; expectorants such as elecampane, hyssop, mullein, and thyme; antiseptic herbs for the respiratory system such as aniseed, garlic, hyssop, oregano, and thyme; and warming herbs like cinnamon, cloves, garlic, ginger, or cayenne pepper. These herbs can be used in teas, giving ½ cup every few hours, or as tinctures or glycerites, giving ½ teaspoon every few hours.

When the cough becomes more pronounced and spastic, use antispasmodic herbs like catnip, crampbark, hyssop, lobelia, or valerian root.

The following herbs are often best given in tincture or glycerite form in small (10 to 30 drops) hourly doses. Try one of these combinations:

Equal parts valerian and chamomile.
Two parts crampbark, one part lobelia, and ½ part peppermint.
Equal parts hyssop, lobelia, and catnip.

Antispasmodic Cough Syrup
Mix in a 4-ounce bottle:

1 oz. garlic syrup
½ oz. catnip glycerite
½ oz. thyme tincture or syrup
½ oz. hyssop tincture
½ oz. crampbark tincture
½ oz. wild lettuce tincture
¼ oz. ginger syrup
¼ oz. elecampane tincture

Give ½ to 1 teaspoon, every 2 hours.

Topical

The regular use of steams, inhalants, and chest rubs can be useful in relaxing the respiratory muscles, increasing the blood flow to the chest, and supporting the immune system.

- Chest rubs increase circulation and warm and relax the chest and respiratory muscles. They are best applied topically before bed or napping. Then cover the chest with a cotton T-shirt. Rubs usually contain aromatic herbs such as eucalyptus, hyssop, thyme, peppermint, camphor, or rosemary, which are very volatile and therefore penetrate the skin easily, stimulate blood flow, relax the muscles, and deliver medication to the local area. They can be especially effective with spastic, tight coughs.
- Herbal steams deliver the medication to the local area. Again, the aromatic, volatile herbs are used. They are all very antiseptic and help to disinfect the respiratory passages. A favorite steam is a combination of 1 teaspoon each of chamomile flowers, yarrow flowers, and lavender flowers.

- Humidify the room, and put hyssop, peppermint, eucalyptus, or yarrow oil in the humidifier as an antispasmodic.
- Use hydrotherapy by trying the wet sock treatment. After thoroughly warming the feet, put cold, damp socks on and cover them with warm, dry wool socks. Have the child sleep with the socks on. This will lessen congestion.

What to Do if Your Child Has Been Exposed

Naturopathic physicians may prescribe pertussis, a homeopathic nosode remedy, to help prevent or ameliorate symptoms. Give 3 to 5 pellets under the tongue once daily, away from other foods or drinks, from the time of exposure for fourteen days. If pertussis develops, consult a physician about whether to use the nosode (and at what frequency) or another homeopathic remedy. Build your child's immune system. Reduce your child's intake of sugar in all forms, as it suppresses the immune system.

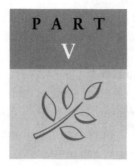

The Child's
Herbal Medicine Chest

See Part VI for instructions on how to make the recommended herbal preparations.

ANISE *Pimpinella anisum*

Part used: Seeds

Actions: Antinausea, antiseptic, antispasmodic, carminative, expectorant, galactagogue

Uses:
Aniseed tea or extracts are very pleasant tasting and easy to give to a child. The herb may be used in all types of cough or lung remedies. It acts as an antiseptic to the respiratory tract's mucous membranes and relaxes the respiratory muscles. I often mix it with thyme, mullein, and elecampane for coughs.

Like fennel seed, aniseed is also used for all types of digestive complaints. It aids in reducing nausea, colic, gas, and spasms in the digestive tract. Simply chewing a few seeds will relieve indigestion.

Preparations and dosages:
Infusion: Use 1 teaspoon to 8 ounces of boiling water. Cover
and steep for 5 minutes. Use ½ to 1 cup, 3 times a day. For
infants, use 1 to 2 droppersful, 3 times a day.
Tincture: Use ½ teaspoon, 3 times a day. For infants, use 5 to
10 drops in a little water, 3 times a day.
Glycerite: Use 1 teaspoon in warm water to make a warm sweet
drink. Take 1 to 3 times a day.

ASHWAGANDHA   *Withania somnifera*

Part used: Root

Actions: Adaptogen, immune modulator, anti-inflammatory,
mild sedative, tonic

Uses:
Adaptogens work to increase the body's ability to cope with
stress. They help to conserve energy. This plant has a mild sedative action that helps to calm the body systems and emotions
while aiding the body in coping with the effects of stress. Use this
plant during times of increased stress or following stressful periods, as it can minimize the effects. It will act to build up the debilitated endocrine, nervous, and immune systems, making it
particularly useful for rehabilitating after long-term stress, including physical trauma and severe illness. It has been shown to promote growth in young children and has an antianemic action.
Often, weight loss and failure to grow are accompanying signs
of stress in a child. This herb is a good specific remedy for such
a child. Use it in combination with licorice root and eleutherococcus for support during and after stressful times, accidents,

emotional trauma, and serious long-term illness. Combine with gingerroot for the anti-inflammatory action to use to combat allergies, joint swelling, sprains, or hives.

Preparations and dosages:

Decoction: The root of the herb can be prepared by using the dry root in a decoction and given as a tea. Since the root does not have the best flavor, I would suggest using it in a blend of roots and seeds to improve the taste. Use a combination of equal amounts of ashwagandha root, licorice root, aniseed, and cinnamon bark. Give the tea warm and sweeten with honey if preferred. Use 1 to 3 cups, daily.

Tincture: Use ¼ to ½ teaspoon of a 1 to 5 strength tincture, 1 to 3 times a day.

ASTRAGALUS *Astragalus membranaceus*

Part used: Root

Actions: Immunostimulate, immunotonic, cardotonic, diuretic, hypotensive.

Uses:

Astragalus is a traditional Chinese medicinal plant that has strong immunomodulating activity. The plant's active chemical constituents act to enhance natural killer cells and increase white blood cell immune activity. Oral doses given over several months have been shown to increase immune substances in nasal secretions, antibody levels, and increased lymphocytes. You can see why this medicinal root makes such an excellent immune system tonic and stimulator.

Traditionally, this plant was used as a tonic to build up the vital response of the body. In a more modern approach it is viewed as an adaptogen, enhancing cell growth, metabolism, memory, longevity, immunity, and resistance. I use this root to help build up the immune system in chronic disease, allergies, and recurring infection, not as much for its stimulating effect, but for its strengthening and building qualities. I combine it with nettles, licorice, and calendula flowers for long-term immune building.

Astragalus root is very useful in supporting body tissues, blood cells, bone marrow, and the immune system in patients receiving chemotherapy and radiation. I suggest giving 4 to 6 capsules daily for this purpose. I would also give this herb for anemias and blood disorders.

Preparations and dosages:

Decoction: Use 1 teaspoon to 8 ounces of cold water. Simmer for 10 to 15 minutes and strain. Use ½ to 1 cup, 3 times a day.

Tincture: Use ½ teaspoon, 3 times a day.

Glycerite: Use 20 to 40 drops, 3 times a day with infants. Use ½ to 1 teaspoon, 3 times a day with older children.

Capsules: Use 2 to 6 per day, depending on age.

CALENDULA *Calendula officinalis*

Part used: Flowers

Actions: Anti-inflammatory, antifungal, antiseptic, cholagogue, diaphoretic, depurative, styptic, vulnerary, stimulates lymphatic system, heals a variety of skin conditions

Uses:

Calendula flowers are well-known for their use in skin and body products. They are soothing, healing, and tonifying to the skin. They inhibit inflammation and promote the growth of new tissue. Calendula flowers are used as lotions, creams, compresses, and oils for inflammation of the skin and mucous membranes, and for healing wounds, boils, bruises, and skin rashes. Use as a gargle for gum, mouth, and throat inflammations and infections; as a wash for leg ulcers, burns, and skin rash; and as a cream for diaper rash, bug bites, and burns. This herb has an antibacterial effect on staphylococcus aureus, a common bacteria responsible for causing many skin infections, including boils, impetigo, and diaper rash. I suggest making an all-purpose calendula salve (see page 262) and keeping it around for general use for cuts, scratches, bites, hemorrhoids, and chapped lips. An infusion of calendula flowers can be used as a hair and scalp rinse for dandruff, itchy scalp, and general health. Calendula may be combined with eyebright in an infusion for an eyewash to soothe and heal red and irritated eyes.

Internally, calendula mildly cleanses the body by stimulating digestion, the lymphatic system, and the liver. It is useful in treating eczema, allergy, and chronic respiratory infection. It stimulates the immune system in a general way to increase white blood cell activity and lymphatic activity. Use with echinacea, wild indigo, and cleavers for tonsillitis, enlarged neck lymph nodes, and pharyngitis. Calendula has a mild, bitter action on the digestive system, thus stimulating digestive secretions and bile, thereby increasing the healing of the digestive mucous membranes. Mix calendula flowers with licorice root and marshmallow root for burning or inflamed stomach or intestines as in diarrhea or after food poisoning.

Many lovely baby skin and bath products are made with calendula flowers, including soaps and shampoos for washing baby, powder for diapering, and salves and creams for skin irritations and cuts. You can also make your own. (See Recipes and Remedies for Infants and Children, starting on page 265.)

Preparations and dosages:
Infusion: Use 1 teaspoon flowers to 8 ounces of boiling water.
Cover and steep for 3 to 5 minutes. Give ½ cup, 3 times a day.

Tincture: Use 30 to 40 drops, 3 times a day. Dilute with water to make an effective antiseptic wash solution for fungal infections of the skin such as ringworm and athlete's foot or cuts and scrapes.

Juice: Fresh calendula juice can be preserved with 25 percent of its weight in alcohol or 50 percent of its weight in vegetable glycerine. Give ½ teaspoon, 3 times a day.

Topical uses: Powdered flowers can be used as a skin and body powder for diaper rash, candida rash, or as a foot powder. Creams and salves can be used topically several times a day for burns, cuts, bites, stings, bruises, skin rash, sunburn, and dry skin. Use the flowers for footbaths, poultices, compresses, and body oils topically as needed for healing and regeneration of tissues.

CATNIP *Nepeta cateria*

Part used: Whole herb

Actions: Antispasmodic, carminative, diaphoretic, febrifuge, relaxant, mild sedative

Uses:

Many people are surprised to learn that catnip is an effective herb for humans. It happens to affect the human nervous system as well as the cat's. Catnip relaxes body tissues and releases tension in the muscles and digestive tract. It has a mild sedating effect on the brain, bringing sleep and quieting the thoughts. It can be mixed with chamomile, lemon balm, and hops for restlessness and insomnia and with meadowsweet, wintergreen, and lemon balm for headache and muscle tension. Mix it with fennel seed and crampbark for relaxing stomach or bowel cramps. It is a favorite choice for colicky babies when mixed with fennel seed and used as a tea to relieve pain and move gas along. This tea also may be helpful in relieving the constipation of infants. Think of catnip for any digestive complaints associated with nervousness, stress, or anxiety. A nice tea blend would be equal amounts of catnip, lemon balm, oats, hops, and cinnamon bark.

Catnip is a good fever remedy, cooling the body by promoting sweating. It also works to cool a fever when taken as a bath or enema. Combine it with elder flowers, yarrow flowers, or meadowsweet in a hot tea for colds and fevers.

Catnip can be applied topically to hemorrhoids as a salve or as a warm compress for tight muscles and headache. Use as a body oil for nerve pain and muscle spasm.

Preparations and dosages:

Infusion: Use 1 teaspoon to 8 ounces of boiling water. Cover and steep for 3 to 5 minutes, and strain. Use ½ cup, 3 times a day. For infants use 1 to 2 droppersful, 3 times a day.

Tincture: Use ½ teaspoon, 3 times a day.

Enema: Use a warm infusion as a rectal enema to bring down fever in a baby or for constipation. With infants, a bulb syringe with an oiled tip makes the perfect-sized enema bag. (See Fever, page 127.)

CHAMOMILE *Matricaria recutita*

Part used: Flowers

Actions: Relaxant, antispasmodic, anodyne, anti-inflammatory, antiseptic, antidiarrheal, antiemetic, carminative, antimicrobial, bitter, vulnerary

Uses:

Chamomile is a wonderful herb for children. It is very gentle in its action yet very effective. This herb is known for its calming effect on the nerves and relaxing effects on the body. It can be used for restlessness, irritability, insomnia, anxiety, and agitation. Chamomile's antispasmodic action makes it useful in treating all types of muscle cramps and spasms. The herb's relaxing qualities also affect the organs of the digestive system, making it especially useful in all types of stomach cramps, colic, constipation, and other digestive upsets caused by tension and anxiety. It is not unusual for children to get a tummyache when tense or emotionally upset.

Chamomile used as an infusion acts quickly to reduce pain, relieve gas, and settle the stomach. The plant contains volatile oils that have an anti-inflammatory action in the stomach and intestines and help to heal the tissue lining the digestive tract. This makes chamomile very useful in the healing of ulcers of the digestive tract. It is also helpful in reducing nausea and vomiting when given in teaspoon doses every few minutes.

Used as a steam, the vapors can be inhaled through the nose into the upper respiratory passages where the herb acts as an antimicrobial, reducing infection and inflammation. It also serves to break up and move out excessive mucus in that area, making the plant useful in treating colds, sinusitis, and hay fever.

Creams, ointments, and washes can be used topically for ezcema, diaper rash, burns, and bruises. A bath of infused flowers can help to calm a nervous or restless child. A wash of the tea can be used for skin irritations, burns, and bug bites.

Preparations and dosages:
Infusion: Use 1 to 2 teaspoons of the dry herb to 8 ounces of
   boiling water. Steep 3 to 5 minutes. Use 1 to 3 cups a day,
   in 1 teaspoon to ½ cup doses.
Tincture: Use ½ to 1 teaspoon, 3 times a day.
Glycerite: Use ½ to 1 teaspoon, 3 times a day.
Steam: Put 1 tablespoon flowers in a large bowl. Pour 1 pint of
   boiling water over the flowers. Make a tent by placing a
   bath towel over the child's head and the bowl and have the

child inhale the steam for 3 to 10 minutes.

Topical uses: Use 1 tablespoon to 1 pint water to make a strong infusion and strain into the bath. Use on the skin as needed.

Herbal pillow: Sew a small 4-inch square pillow and stuff with chamomile flowers; place in the child's bed to aid sleep and discourage bad dreams. (See Sleeplessness/Insomnia, page 170.)

CINNAMON *Cinnamomum* spp.

Part used: Bark

Actions: Antimicrobial, antispasmodic, antidiarrheal, anthelmintic, carminative, circulatory stimulant, refrigerant

Uses:

This warming spice makes a pleasant-tasting remedy to soothe the stomach and decrease gas, indigestion, colic, and nausea. It can be taken as a tea or used in tincture form for stomach upset, belching, lack of appetite, diarrhea, or stomach cramps. Mix ½ teaspoon each of cinnamon and unsweetened carob powder in 2 tablespoons of applesauce; give several times a day for diarrhea. Add cinnamon to flu and fever teas to keep the fever in check and for its antimicrobial effect in fighting influenza infection. A good combination would be equal amounts of cinnamon bark, linden flowers, yarrow flowers, and peppermint given as a tea or tincture.

Cinnamon tincture mixed with garlic syrup, wormwood, black walnut, and sage tinctures can be used for intestinal worms. Use ½ teaspoon, 3 times a day, for 7 days and repeat in 2 weeks.

Preparations and dosages:

Decoction: Use 1 teaspoon dried bark to 8 ounces of water. Cover, simmer for 10 minutes, and strain. Use ½ cup, 3 times a day.

Tincture: Use ¼ teaspoon in a little water, 3 times a day. I seldom use cinnamon tincture alone. Usually I mix one part of tincture to other herbs in a formula.

Glycerite: Use ½ teaspoon, 3 times a day, in a cup of warm water to make a sweet warm drink. This makes a great addition to cold and cough formula, bringing a warming quality and improving the taste.

CLEAVERS *Galium aparine*

Part used: Whole herb

Actions: Alterative, astringent, diuretic, vulnerary

Uses:

This plant is also known as goosegrass because of its rough stems, which catch you as you walk by. Cleavers is a major remedy influencing the lymphatic system. A fresh juice or fresh tincture will increase lymphatic circulation, increase lymph node drainage, and reduce lymphatic swelling. Include this herb in formulas for ear infections, tonsillitis, upper respiratory infection, and urinary infection. Cleavers can be taken safely over a period of time to soften and decrease enlarged lymph nodes or for treating eczema or psoriasis.

Cleavers increases urine flow, soothes the urinary tract, and reduces inflammation. Combine it with urinary antiseptics like thyme or uva ursi for cystitis or urinary tract infections. Give it hourly as a tea.

Fresh cleavers herb is far superior to the dry herb, as drying, storage, and heat all decrease its medicinal potency. Juice the herb and preserve it with 25 percent its weight in alcohol or 50 percent its weight in vegetable glycerine. The fresh juice may also be frozen in ice cube trays and defrosted as needed.

Cleavers poultice made from the pulverized fresh herb can be applied over enlarged swollen glands and lymph nodes. Creams and salves can be made to use topically for swellings, skin rash, bites, or burns.

Preparations and dosages:

Infusion: Use 2 teaspoons to 8 ounces of boiling water. Steep for 5 minutes and strain. Use 1 cup, 3 times a day.

Tincture: Use ½ teaspoon, 3 times a day. Use tinctures made from the fresh herb only.

Glycerite: Use 1 teaspoon, 3 times a day. Cleavers extracts well in glycerine or use it to preserve the fresh juice.

Poultice: Chop, puree, or macerate fresh cleavers, apply to area, and cover with gauze. Leave on for 20 minutes.

CONEFLOWER *Echinacea* spp.

Parts used: Root (*E. augustifolia*); whole herb and root (*E. purpurea*); whole herb and root (*E. pallida*)

Actions: Antiseptic, antimicrobial, antiviral, immune stimulant, vulnerary

Uses:

This medicinal plant was highly valued by Native Americans. It was used to treat fevers, snakebites, wounds, toothaches, and infections. Today, it is one of the most researched and studied medicinal herbs and has been shown to have many valued pharmaceutical actions. All varieties of echinacea have been shown to affect the immune system in diverse ways such as stimulating nonspecific immune responses; increasing white blood cell and lymphocyte activity at the site of infection; increasing production of white blood cells; and enhancing the ability of some white blood cells to eat up foreign substances such as bacteria, fungus, and virus. The fresh juice of *E. purpurea* has antiviral activity against herpes and influenza.

The coneflower has gained popularity because of its well-publicized ability to boost the immune system and fight infection. There are hundreds of echinacea products on the market. Some are blends of different plant parts and/or plant species. Most of the research on echinacea's effects on the immune system have been on *E. purpurea*, though *E. augustifolia* was the species traditionally used. *E. augustifolia* has been overharvested in the United States and is becoming threatened. Many growers are cultivating this plant to ensure its availability. I often choose to use a combination of the whole herb of *E. purpurea* and *E. augustifolia* root in the same preparation.

For acute types of infections like ear infection, respiratory infection, sinusitis, influenza, stomach flu, or urinary tract or kidney infection, use echinacea in larger doses and more frequently. I suggest ½ teaspoon, 4 or 5 times a day for the most acute part of the illness. Then, as the child is improving, lower the dose to 3 times a day and continue for another week after the symptoms have gone.

If a child has recurring infections, such as chronic ear infections, I would suggest using a low dose of echinacea on a daily basis over an extended time. Often, I mix it for this purpose with astragalus, elder flowers, nettles, and ginger. If an ear infection occurs, I stop using the formula for daily use and use echinacea alone at ½ teaspoon, 4 or 5 times daily, as described above for acute infection.

Echinacea tea can be used daily for cleansing the lymphatic system and skin. I find it helpful with boils, acne, ringworm, herpes, and warts. It makes a great throat and mouthwash for infected gums, throat, tonsillitis, laryngitis, and mouth ulcers. Topically, a wash can be used on wounds, skin infections, and bug bites. I often mix it with myrrh, tea tree oil, and calendula flowers as a footbath for athlete's foot or as a rinse for any fungal infection.

Preparations and dosages:

Decoction of the root: Use 1 teaspoon to 8 ounces of water. Simmer for 10 minutes and strain. Use 1 cup, 3 times a day.

Infusion of whole herb: Use 2 teaspoons to 8 ounces of boiling water. Steep for 5 to 10 minutes and strain. Take 1 cup, 3 times a day.

Tincture: Use ½ to 1 teaspoon, 3 times a day. For infants, use 20 to 40 drops, 3 times a day.

Juice: Use ½ to 1 teaspoon, 3 times a day. For infants, use 20 to 40 drops.

Capsules: Use 250 to 500 milligrams, 3 times a day.

Standardized extract: Use 100 to 250 milligrams, 3 times a day.

Topical uses: The powdered herb can be used as a wound powder or nasal snuff. Or it can be mixed with water to a paste and applied to boils. It can also be used as a wash, compress, cream, or salve.

ELDER *Sambucus nigra* and species

Parts used: Flowers, berries

Actions: Anticatarrhal, diaphoretic, stimulates nonspecific immune function

Uses:

Elder, a low-growing shrub, has two medicinally active parts: the flowers and the berries. The dark purple berries are high in flavonoid compounds, which have therapeutic activity as antiviral, anti-inflammatory, antioxidant, and immunotonic agents.

The flowers stimulate nonspecific immune function particularly in the upper respiratory system, nasal mucosa, and sinuses. Traditionally, they have been used to tonify and strengthen the mucous membranes, making this botanical medicine useful in the treatment of acute and chronic respiratory diseases.

Make a syrup of elderberry by using 2 cups fresh elderberries to 1 cup raw sugar or ¾ cup of pure vegetable glycerin. Combine the berries and sugar and slowly heat to a simmer for 3 minutes. Remove from the heat, mash with potato masher, and steep warm mix for 30 minutes. Puree, strain, and bottle. Use ½ to 1 teaspoon per dose, 3 times a day. This is an excellent base for mixing other immune-boosting and antiviral tinctures to make them more palatable for small children. Keep in the refrigerator when storing for longer than 2 months.

Preparations and dosages:
Infusion: Use 1 teaspoon herb to 8 ounces of boiling water.
Steep for 5 minutes and strain. Drink ½ to 1 cup, 3 times a day. Give 1 to 2 droppersful, per dose, to an infant.
Tincture: Use ½ to 1 teaspoon, 3 times a day.
Glycerite: Use 1 teaspoon, 3 times a day. Add to warm water to make a sweet warm drink.
Topical uses: A wash of elder flowers can be used to cool fevers, stop skin itching, and dry up sores. Add the infusion to a warm bath to bring down fevers.

ELECAMPANE   *Inula helenium*

Part used: Root

Actions: Antitussive, anthelmintic, bitter, expectorant

Uses:
Elecampane is an excellent choice for relieving coughs when they are dry, irritated, and nonproductive. The root of the plant increases the watery secretion of the respiratory system, making the cough productive and less irritating. This plant also decreases spasms of the chest, making it useful in treating bronchitis, asthma, and bronchial pneumonia. The root acts as a mild bitter, slightly stimulating the appetite and bowels. I like to include it in respiratory combinations to support digestion. The root has mild antimicrobial qualities due to the small amount of volatile oils, making it a useful remedy for pinworms and parasites.

Preparations and dosages:
Decoction: Soak 1 ounce of the root in 1 pint of water for 1 hour. Bring to a boil and simmer 10 to 15 minutes. Take 1 cup, twice a day.
Tincture or glycerite: Use ½ to 1 teaspoon, 3 times a day.

EYEBRIGHT *Euphrasia officinalis*

Part used: Whole herb

Actions: Anticatarrhal, anti-inflammatory, astringent, local soothing action on the eye

Uses:
As the name suggests, this plant is used for the eyes. It may be taken internally for strengthening the eyes and relieving allergic eye symptoms. An herb infusion can be used as an eyewash for irritations, conjunctivitis, styes, and eye infections. The tannins in the plant have an astringent effect on the eye membrane and reduce inflammation.

Eyebright has a restoring, healing, and strengthening action on the mucous membranes of the eyes, nose, throat, and sinuses. It regulates mucous secretions and stops overproduction by constricting the nasal membranes. I find it useful for a chronic runny nose, allergic sinusitis, fluid in the ear, and postnasal drip. I often combine it with elder flowers, ribwort, and fenugreek seed. Use eyebright daily for several months to help restore the mucous membranes.

Preparations and dosages:
Infusion: Use 1 teaspoon of the herb to 8 ounces of boiling water. Steep for 3 to 5 minutes and strain. Use ½ to 1 cup, 3 times a day.
Tincture: Use ½ teaspoon, 3 times a day, in water or juice.
Glycerite: Use 1 teaspoon, 3 times a day, in warm water.
Topical uses: Soak a cloth in an infusion of the herb and apply over the eyes for swollen or sore eyes. Use as an eyewash for infections and pink eye.

FENNEL *Foeniculum vulgare*

Part used: Seed

Actions: Anti-inflammatory, bronchodilator, carminative, diuretic, galactagogue, mild laxative

Uses:
Fennel seed is a pleasant-tasting herb that relieves colic, gas, and discomfort in the digestive tract. Fennel acts as a mild laxative and intestinal relaxant, easing tension from the colon wall. It is excellent for colicky babies. Fennel tea can be added to the formula, a dropperful can be given directly to the baby, or a breast-feeding mother can drink the tea and pass it along to the infant in her milk. Fennel tea may be used for constipation, gas, nausea, and vomiting. Fennel seed should always be added to laxative formulas for children, as it will prevent cramping of the bowel. One of my favorite combinations for stomach cramps is fennel, lemon balm, and catnip tea.

Fennel is also good to use to treat respiratory infections and coughs, as it not only relaxes and decreases bronchial spasms but also has an antimicrobial action due to the excretion of its volatile oil into the lungs. The pleasant taste of the tincture or syrup makes it easy to give.

An infusion of the seeds can be used as an eyewash for styes, conjunctivitis, or itchy eyes. Fennel tea makes a healing mouth-wash for sore gums and throats. Combine it with equal parts of thyme and peppermint.

Preparations and dosages:
Infusion: Use 1 teaspoon of the seeds to 8 ounces of boiling
water. Cover and steep for 35 minutes. Use ½ to 1 cup, 3
times a day. For infants, use 1 to 2 droppersful, 3 times a day.
Due to the high volatile oil content of fennel seed, an infusion
rather than a decoction is used to avoid loss of the oil.

Tincture: Use ½ teaspoon, 3 times a day. For infants use 5 to 10 drops in a little water, 3 times a day.

Glycerite: Use ½ to 1 teaspoon, 3 times a day. This can be added to warm water to make a sweet hot drink.

Chew the fresh seeds to relieve indigestion, heartburn, gas, or bad breath.

GARLIC *Allium sativum*

Parts used: Bulb or cloves

Actions: Antimicrobial, anticoagulant, antihistaminic, anti-hypertensive, anthelmintic, antitoxin, expectorant, lowers blood cholesterol levels, regulates blood sugar

Uses:

Garlic has a long history of medicinal use. Probably one of the most popular is its ability to fight infections caused by bacteria, viruses, parasites, or fungi. Garlic is particularly useful in all types of infections of the nose, sinuses, throat, and lungs. This is not only because of garlic's immune-boosting effects but also because of the sulfur-containing compounds found in garlic that are taken out of the body through the lungs. This allows its antimicrobial action to help heal the respiratory system. Garlic also has a strong effect on digestive infections such as worms, parasites, candida, viruses, and bacteria. For respiratory infections take garlic raw, in syrups, capsules, honey, tinctures, or juice. Garlic syrup is a great base for tinctures and glycerites. Garlic oil may be used warm in the ear for ear infections and earache.

Garlic has a beneficial effect on the heart and the blood vessels and makes an excellent long-term remedy for the cardiovascular system. Garlic dilates the blood vessels in the peripheral circulation and lowers blood pressure. It has also been effective in lowering cholesterol levels in the blood and reducing the risk of atherosclerosis in adults.

When taken regularly in the diet, garlic also regulates blood sugar metabolism. This makes the plant useful in the treatment of hypoglycemia in children.

Garlic may be used topically in oils and salves, or it may be used fresh. When using fresh garlic put a little oil on the skin before applying the garlic to avoid burning or blistering the skin. Use garlic juice on infected wounds, as a gargle for throat infections, or as a poultice for warts.

Preparations and dosages:
Freshly minced garlic can be swallowed whole with water or juice for coughs, bronchitis, pneumonia, pinworms, or parasites.

Garlic Syrup
10 to 12 cloves of garlic, sliced
1 cup raw sugar

Layer sugar and slices of garlic in a glass jar. Let sit in a cool place for 1 to 2 days, strain out the garlic, and bottle in an amber jar. Use ½ to 1 teaspoon, 3 times a day. Can be added to warm tea.

Garlic Honey
Slice 6 cloves of garlic and add to 4 ounces of honey. Let stand for 7 to 10 days. Use the garlic honey in medicinal teas for colds, flu, sore throat, cough, or sinusitis. The garlic cloves may be eaten on toast or crackers.

Garlic Oil
Slice 6 to 8 cloves of fresh garlic and cover in a jar with 4 ounces of olive oil. Steep for 7 days, strain, and pour into a dark bottle. Use as an ear oil, chest rub, or on wounds.

GINGER   *Zingiber officinale*

Part used: Root

Actions: Anti-inflammatory, antinausea, carminative, circulatory stimulant, diaphoretic, antispasmodic

Uses:
The pungent taste of this spice makes it very warming to the body, increasing blood flow and warming the digestive tract. It has been shown to be an effective remedy against the nausea of pregnancy, motion sickness, and postoperation. Before traveling, 1 or 2 capsules can reduce travel sickness. I often mix ⅓ ounce of ginger tincture with ⅔ ounce of distilled water in a 1-ounce dropper bottle, dosing 1 to 2 droppersful as needed for symptoms of nausea and vomiting. The volatile oils in ginger gently stimulate digestive secretions and the muscles of the digestive tract.

Ginger's anti-inflammatory action inhibits synthesis of inflammatory substances in the body, making it useful in treating inflammation of the joints, skin, lungs, and digestive tract. I include ginger in many formulas, as it increases blood flow to tissues and helps to bring the other herbal components of the formula to the site that needs healing. It warms up chills, stabilizes fevers, and quiets cough spasms. A dash of dried powder can be added to any herbal tea, or 10 to 15 drops of ginger tincture can be added to any 1-ounce tincture formula. Ginger syrup makes a great addition to teas, cough syrups, and sparkling water. New Chapter Extracts of Brattleboro, Vermont, makes an excellent Ginger Wonder Syrup.

Preparations and dosages:
Decoction: Use 4 to 5 slices of fresh root or ½ teaspoon of dried cut root to 8 ounces of water. Simmer for 10 minutes and strain. Use 1 tablespoon to ½ cup, 3 times a day.
Tincture: Use 2 to 10 drops in a little water or juice.

Glycerite: Use 5 to 15 drops in a little water.

Compress: A ginger compress can be used on the chest or upper back to break up congestion and bring blood into the lung area when treating pneumonia or bronchitis. (See Recipes and Remedies for Infants and Children, starting on page 265.)

Fresh Ginger Vegetable Juice
5 carrots
1 apple
½ inch of fresh gingerroot

Juice ingredients together in a vegetable juicer. Some children may prefer this diluted with a little water.

HOPS *Humulus lupulus*

Part used: Strobiles

Actions: Aromatic bitter, sedative, antispasmodic, soporific

Uses:

There are two conditions for which I use hops for children. The first is for a sluggish, nervous digestion that may be accompanied by pain in the tummy. Often, with tension or stress, digestion slows down and weakens. Hops gently stimulates the digestive function and regulates the appetite. Its antispasmodic action relaxes the smooth muscle and reduces pain and discomfort. If the child will not take a hops tea, then a warm compress soaked in the tea and applied to the stomach with extra heat from a hot water bottle will work nicely. Second, I use hops with children who struggle with sleeplessness, excitability, and restlessness. A warm hops bath taken before bed will help to quiet the child, or a pillow stuffed with lavender and hops tucked inside the child's sleeping pillow can gently lull the child off to sleep. I often mix hops with other herbs like lavender, linden flowers, catnip, chamomile, or skullcap when treating restlessness, excitability, and hyperactivity in children.

Preparations and dosages:

Infusion: Use 1 teaspoon of the herb to 1 cup boiling water. Steep for 1 to 3 minutes and strain. Give ¼ to 1 cup, 3 times a day.

Tincture: For ages 6 to 24 months, use 5 to 15 drops, 3 times a day. For ages 3 to 10 years, use 20 to 60 drops, 3 times a day.

Topical uses: Use the warm infusion as a skin wash for wounds and skin infections.

HYSSOP *Hyssopus officinalis*

Part used: Whole herb

Actions: Antimicrobial, antifungal, antibacterial, antispasmodic, carminative, expectorant, relaxant

Uses:

This aromatic member of the mint family has a strong effect on the lungs and respiratory muscles. It relaxes the bronchioles and muscles of the chest, making it especially useful in treating spastic coughs, asthma, and whooping cough. It is one of the primary herbs that I choose for the treatment of whooping cough. I suggest it be used as an herbal tincture, given as a hot tea, or used as an essential oil for steam inhalation. It is often best to give the tea with a little honey, as it can taste bitter. Have the child sip the tea from a teaspoon over time. This way the stomach will not become too full, which can lead to gagging when having a coughing spell. Hyssop makes a good antiseptic gargle for sore throat or laryngitis. It is also helpful in the treatment of fevers that are associated with colds and coughs. Hyssop cools the body by producing a sweat and fighting the infection. I like to mix it with herbs like elder flowers, meadowsweet, yarrow, or linden flowers. Like the herb thyme, hyssop has an antiseptic action on the urinary system, making this tea useful in the treatment of cystitis. Topically, I like to use the plant in antifungal skin washes, ointments, and creams against candida rash, tinea, and boils.

Preparations and dosages:

Infusion: Add 1 teaspoon of the herb to 1 cup of boiling water. Cover and steep for 1 to 3 minutes. It is best to sweeten with honey or fruit juice, or mix with other pleasant-tasting herbs such as licorice, aniseed or spearmint.

Tincture or glycerite: Use ½ to 1 teaspoon, 3 times a day.

Chest rub: Use 5 drops of essential oil in 1 ounce of olive oil. Apply to chest and back area to break up congestion.

Hyssop can also be used in footbaths, steams, creams, and ointments.

LAVENDER *Lavendula officinalis*

Part used: Flowers

Actions: Analgesic, antidepressant, antispasmodic, carminative

Uses:

The pleasant scent of lavender is well-known and widely used in cosmetics. This plant is also a valued medicinal herb used as a relaxant to decrease tension in the body and to quiet the mind. It is especially useful in treating headaches and upset stomach due to nervousness, tension, or excitability. It can be taken as a tea, tincture, or bath depending on age and compliance. The aromatic scent has a calming effect on the nervous system and can be used in a pillow for inducing sleep. A drop of lavender oil put on a warm lightbulb will fill the air with its wonderfully calming scent. The oil also has antiseptic qualities, which make the herb very useful in the topical treatment of skin infections, boils, and cuts. Used as a steam inhalant, it soothes and disinfects the passages of the nose, sinuses, and upper throat. A body oil made from lavender will relieve pain in the nerves, muscles, ligaments, and joints. Ground to a fine powder and sifted, the flowers make a wonderful addition to baby powders.

The essential oil of this herb has an uplifting effect on one's emotional state and mood. The aroma of the herb affects the mood center of the brain by stimulating the nerves in the nose.

Preparations and dosages:

Infusion: Use 1 teaspoon to 1 cup of boiling water; cover, steep for 3 to 5 minutes, and strain. Give ½ to 1 cup, 3 times day.

Tincture or glycerite: Use 5 to 30 drops, 3 times a day.

Topical uses: Use as a body powder, skin wash, body oil, cream, or ointment. Lavender water makes an excellent skin wash for the treatment of acne and boils.

Essential oil: Use 1 to 3 drops in hot water as a steam inhalant for nasal congestion and sinus headache. Use a few drops in the bath for muscle or joint pain or to quiet the mind and lift the spirits.

LEMON BALM *Melissa officinalis*

Part used: Leaves

Actions: Antispasmodic, antiviral, antidepressant, carminative, circulatory stimulant, diaphoretic, nervine

Uses:

The lemon-scented volatile oils of this plant are responsible for many of lemon balm's medicinal actions. The pure essential oil used as a steam inhalant acts as an antimicrobial in the respiratory tract and stimulates the secretions of the membranes. The scent of the oils has a calming, relaxing, and mood-elevating effect on the nervous system by stimulating the limbic or pleasure centers of the brain directly through the olfactory nerves in the nose. A few drops can be diffused in boiling water or dabbed on a lightbulb to release the pleasant scent.

Teas and tinctures of lemon balm are useful in treating fevers, flu, respiratory infections, and digestive complaints. A lemon balm tea is especially good when a child has a flu with fever and nausea. Give the tea freely throughout the day by the tablespoon. For nervous or upset stomach due to anxiety, emotional upset, or indigestion, use 5 to 10 drops of the tincture in a little water or in a warm tea. This gentle herb stimulates digestive function, reduces gas and bloating, and releases tension from the digestive tract muscles and organs.

For digestive discomfort due to cramping, bloating, constipation, or food poisoning, I often use lemon balm in a mix with crampbark, catnip, and meadowsweet, giving it in tablespoon doses. A member of the mint family, lemon balm contains active constituents called tannins. Tannins help to firm tissue and decrease local irritation. The tannins in this plant make it useful in treating diarrhea, nausea, and topical wounds.

Lemon balm as a tea, tincture, or bath or body rub quiets the mind and body, relaxes the muscles, reduces excitability, and calms the spirit. Include it in remedies for nervousness, anxiety, restlessness, butterflies in the stomach, stage fright, and sadness. A bath of lemon balm, hops, and linden flowers can be used for insomnia and restlessness at night.

Preparations and dosages:

Infusion: Use 1 teaspoon to 8 ounces of boiling water. Steep for 3 to 5 minutes and strain. Give ½ to 1 cup, 3 times a day. For babies, give by the dropperful.

Tincture: Use ½ teaspoon, 3 times a day. For infants, dilute ½ ounce tincture with ½ ounce of water and use 20 to 30 drops per dose.

Topical uses: Use in baths, sleep pillows, compresses, or massage oils. A cream or ointment of lemon balm helps to heal cold sores and herpes.

Essential oil: Use a few drops in a bath or steam for the upper respiratory system or in a body oil. Some children's skin may be sensitive to the essential oil, so test a small spot of skin on the forearm with a dab of oil if your child has skin sensitivities.

LICORICE *Glycyrrhiza glabra*

Part used: Root

Actions: Anti-inflammatory, antiviral, demulcent, expectorant, hypertensive, secretolytic, antispasmodic

Uses:

This sweet-tasting herb has a strong folklore of use as a cough and digestive remedy. Modern scientific research has confirmed its folklore uses and discovered its antiviral and anti-inflammatory properties. The herb is popular with children due to its pleasant taste. The tea makes an excellent throat gargle for sore irritated throats. It soothes dry, spastic coughs and fights viral and bacterial respiratory infections. The tea's sweet taste can help to mask the taste of less palatable herbs.

As a digestive remedy, the plant soothes inflammation of the mucous membranes that line the digestive tract, promoting healing of the digestive mucosal lining and increasing production of the mucosal secretions that aid in protecting the membranes. The most efficient form of licorice root for this purpose is the deglycyrrhizinated licorice, DGL. Research has shown this to be very effective in the treatment of ulcers, colitis, and other gastrointestinal inflammations.

When the licorice root is deglycyrrhizinated it is safe for adult hypertensives, as the active constituent responsible for elevating blood pressure has been removed. Those suffering from hypertension or low potassium levels should avoid using this plant in its whole form whether in tea, tincture, or capsule. Deglycyrrhizinated licorice comes in a chewable tablet that can be used for children with diarrhea, heartburn, or indigestion.

Licorice inhibits viral RNA and DNA, leading to a significant antiviral activity. Licorice also inhibits viral activity by activating natural killer cells and macrophages. Think of this plant when treating any childhood viral diseases such as chicken pox; measles; hand, foot, and mouth disease; herpes simplex, or any acute viral infection.

A topical gel ointment makes an excellent medication for herpes sores, cold sores, or shingles lesions. The gel helps to quiet the itching and dries the sores up quickly.

Preparations and dosages:

Decoction: Use 1 to 2 teaspoons to 8 ounces of water. Simmer for 5 to 10 minutes and strain. Give ½ to 1 cup, 3 times a day.

Tincture: Use ½ to 1 teaspoon, 3 times a day. Use the tincture to flavor other medicines that taste unpleasant.

Capsules: Take 1 capsule, 3 times a day.

Deglycyrrhizinated tablets or capsules: Use 1 capsule, 3 or 4
   times a day before or after food.

Licorice Cough Drops

Make a decoction of 1 ounce of licorice root in 8 ounces of
water. Simmer uncovered for 20 minutes, strain out the
herb, add 4 ounces of raw sugar, and simmer until thick.
Remove from heat and sift in 2 teaspoons of slippery elm
powder while stirring. Mix well and drop by the teaspoonful onto wax paper to cool.

LINDEN (Lime Tree Flowers) *Tillia* spp.

Part used: Flowers

Actions: Astringent, antispasmodic, diaphoretic, diuretic, hypotensive, sedative

Uses:

Linden flowers affect the nervous system by calming irritation,
relaxing the body, and releasing tension. They may be used alone
or in combination with hops, lemon balm, chamomile, or lavender flowers for headaches, migraines, restlessness, and anxiety.
An infusion may be sipped or used in a relaxing bath. I find linden flowers to be helpful in treating influenza. Given as a hot tea
alone or with peppermint and elder flowers helps to resolve the
illness quickly and with fewer complications. The same combination will work in tincture form when ½ teaspoon is given in
warm water. Linden flowers can be used to treat all types of
fevers, helping the body to sweat and cool itself.

Preparations and dosages:

Infusion: Use 1 to 2 teaspoons of the flowers to 8 ounces of boiling water. Cover and steep for 5 minutes. Give ½ to 1 cup, 3 times a day.

Tincture: Use ¼ to ½ teaspoon, 3 times a day.

Bath: Use a strong infusion in a warm bath.

MARSHMALLOW *Althea officinalis*

Parts used: Root and leaves

Actions: Antitussive, demulcent, diuretic, emollient, expectorant, vulnerary

Uses:

This mucilaginous, white-rooted herb tends to soothe inflammation, decrease irritation, and heal any tissues it touches. The mucous membranes of the digestive, respiratory, and urinary systems all benefit from marshmallow's soothing action. A decoction of the root can be used to treat gastritis, diarrhea, ulcer, coughs, sore throats, cystitis, and urinary tract infections. The root makes an effective syrup base for cold and cough remedies.

Instead of using the marshmallow root in cough remedies, the leaves are sometimes used for their stronger expectorant effect on the lungs since there is less mucilage found in the leaf. The leaf can also be added to teas for cystitis.

Topically, marshmallow root soothes irritations such as burns, skin rashes, or bug bites. Used as a poultice, the root draws thorns, splinters, and infections to the surface. The powdered root can be used as a wound powder or baby powder. A salve made from the root can be used on cuts, scratches, boils, burns, bites, stings, and splinters.

Preparations and dosages:

Decoction: Soak 2 tablespoons of the root in 1 pint of cold
water overnight. Simmer for 10 minutes in the morning and
strain out root. Give up to 1 cup, 3 times a day.

Tincture: Use ¼ to ½ teaspoon, 3 times a day.

Topical uses: Use as a soak, poultice, powder, cream, or salve.

Syrup: See Recipes and Remedies for Infants and Children,
starting on page 265.

Cold and Cough Remedy

4 oz. marshmallow syrup (See Recipes and Remedies for
Infants and Children, starting on page 265.)

½ oz. thyme tincture

½ oz. echinacea tincture

½ oz. elder flowers tincture

½ oz. ginger syrup

Mix in a large bottle. Use ½ to 1 teaspoon, 3 or 4 times a
day.

MEADOWSWEET *Filipendula ulmaria*

Part used: Whole herb

Actions: Astringent, analgesic, antacid, anti-inflammatory, antiseptic, diaphoretic, diuretic, digestive aid

Uses:

Meadowsweet makes a nice-tasting tea either as a simple tea or
when mixed with other herbs. It can be combined with lemon
balm and elder flowers for fevers and flus, with aniseed for digestive upset, and with wintergreen for headache or muscle pain.
Slowly sipping 10 drops of the tincture in an ounce of warm
water will reduce nausea or overacidity of the stomach. Com-

bined with uva ursi and cornsilk, meadowsweet is a soothing antiseptic tea for cystitis.

A compress soaked in meadowsweet tea will help to reduce inflammation and relieve joint and nerve pain. An infusion can also be used as an eyewash for conjunctivitis and styes.

Preparations and dosages:

Infusion: Use 1 teaspoon to 1 cup of boiling water. Steep for 3 to 5 minutes and strain. Use 1 to 3 droppersful with infants; 1 to 3 teaspoons with toddlers; and ½ cup with older children, 3 times a day.

Tincture: Use 15 drops with infants and ½ teaspoon with older children, 3 times a day.

MINT: PEPPERMINT *Mentha piperita* and SPEARMINT *Mentha spicata*

Part used: Leaves

Actions: Astringent, antiseptic, antipuritic, antispasmodic, anti-emetic, carminative, diaphoretic, mild bitter

Uses:

I prefer to use spearmint rather than peppermint when working with children because the flavor and actions are milder. In general, I don't recommend using peppermint with babies or for long periods of time with young children. The mints have a strong influence on the digestive tract, relaxing the muscles reducing nausea, vomiting, gas, and bloating. They mildly stimulate digestion making them helpful in relieving the discomfort from overeating or sluggish digestion. I like to have children sip tea-spoon doses for colic, indigestion, flatulence, or nausea. Mint added to cold and flu teas promotes sweating and helps to reduce fever. Because it increases blood circulation, it is also particularly useful for chills. The mints are also known for their relaxing and cooling action when used for treating headaches and migraines. Topically, a mint infusion can be used to cool itchy skin, reduce joint swelling, and reduce the pain of a bug bite or a cold sore. The essential oil of peppermint can be used as an inhalation for nasal and lung congestion. A few drops in a wash relieve skin irritations, burns, itch, inflammations, chicken pox, herpes sores, or ringworm.

Preparations and dosages:
Infusion: Use 1 teaspoon to 8 ounces of boiling water. Cover
  and steep for 3 to 5 minutes. Give 1 cup, 3 times a day.
Tincture or glycerite: Use ¼ to ½ teaspoon, 3 times a day.
Topical uses: Use 1 to 3 drops topically in baths, steams, skin
  washes, or in massage oils, creams, or salves.

MULLEIN *Verbascum thapsus*

Parts used: Leaves and flowers

Actions: Demulcent, emolient, expectorant, vulnerary, mildly antispasmodic, relaxing

Uses:
Mullein is a lovely plant, with its tall stalks of yellow flowers and large, fuzzy green-gray leaves. This plant is essential in the treatment of earaches in children. The flowers are steeped in warm oil and then applied as warm drops into the ear. The plant soothes irritation, relieves inflammation, and brings relief from ear pain and pressure. Other herbs in an oil form, such as St. John's wort, calendula, goldenseal, and garlic, can be mixed with the mullein oil to make an herbal ear drop formula. (See Recipes and Remedies for Infants and Children, starting on page 265.)

Mullein is an excellent medicinal treatment for colds, coughs, bronchitis, and asthma. The herb soothes irritated mucous membranes in the throat and lungs, loosens tight coughs and congestion, and relaxes the muscles of the chest. It also opens the airways and makes breathing easier. It may be given as a tea, tincture, or syrup for coughs and colds; as a gargle with licorice for a dry, irritated throat; or as a hot compress used externally for tonsillitis.

Mullein's anti-inflammatory qualities make it useful in treating bruises and swellings of the glands, muscles, and ligaments. It may be applied over the affected area as a warm compress or in an oil. I often mix in a little lobelia when using it for this purpose. A tincture combining equal parts of the following herbs makes a helpful first-aid formula for sprains, bruises, and bumps: mullein leaves, lobelia, and wormwood. Mix in a bottle, shake well, and apply to the area 3 to 4 times a day.

Preparations and dosages:

Infusion: Use 1 to 2 teaspoons per cup of boiling water. Steep for 3 to 5 minutes, strain, and drink 1 cup, 3 times a day.

Tincture or glycerite: Take ½ teaspoon, 3 times a day, before food.

Topical uses: Use as a compress, footbath, or in body oils. For use as a neck wrap, see Recipes and Remedies for Infants and Children, starting on page 265.

NETTLES *Urtica dioica*

Part used: Leaves

Actions: Astringent, alterative, diuretic, galactagogue, nutritive, septic, tonic

Uses:
Nettles not only have valuable medicinal qualities but also have important nutritional value. This mineral-rich herb pulls minerals from the soil such as iron, potassium, calcium, and zinc. The plant is also high in vitamin C and bioflavonoids. The tender young shoots make an excellent vegetable used as a steamed green or in a soup. The plant has a long history of use as a spring tonic to cleanse and tone the body. A tablespoon of nettle juice taken daily for several weeks works well. The juice can also be used to boost iron levels in iron-deficient anemia and to heal the digestive tract after gastritis or diarrhea.

Medicinally, the herb stimulates the lymph system, affecting the glands and lymph nodes. This makes it useful in swollen glands, enlarged lymph nodes, and infection. Nettles stimulate the flow of urine and reduce fluid retention in the tissues, a useful treatment for edema, cystitis, and water retention. Nettles in the freeze-dried form stabilize histamine response in the body, helping to reduce allergic reaction, hay fever, hives, eczema, and asthma.

A tea may be used regularly to promote health, support waste-removal systems, provide minerals and vitamins, and tonify the tissues. See the recipe for Healthy Herbal Punch for Kids in Part VI (page 273), which I recommend as a winter tonic for wellness.

The tincture may be used to promote mother's milk or to stop bleeding and treat skin conditions.

Topically, an infusion can be used as a wash or compress for cuts, rashes, bug bites, swellings, nerve pain, or sprains or made into a salve or cream for cuts, bug bites, hemorrhoids, or burns.

An infusion of nettles can be used as a hair rinse to treat dandruff or hair loss or as a general rinse for healthy hair. Use as a final rinse and do not rinse out.

Preparations and dosages:

Infusion: Use 1 teaspoon to 8 ounces of boiling water. Steep for 3 to 5 minutes and strain. Give ½ to 1 cup, 3 times a day.

Tincture: Use ¼ to ½ teaspoon, 3 times a day.

Glycerite: Use ½ to 1 teaspoon, 3 times a day.

Juice: Use 1 to 3 teaspoons, 3 times a day. Juice may be stored in the refrigerator for 2 to 3 days. It may be preserved by adding ½ of its weight in vegetable glycerine. Juice may be frozen in ice cube trays and used throughout the winter.

Topical uses: Creams, salves, washes, compresses, poultices, and powders can be used for all types of skin conditions and rashes.

OATS *Avena sativa*

Parts used: Seeds and whole herb

Actions: Antidepressive, cardiac tonic, nutritive, restorative to the nervous system

Uses:

This herb is considered to be one of the major restoratives for the nervous system in the herbal materia medica. In fact, it actually feeds the nervous system. It is especially good for tissue depletion associated with depressive states. This makes oats useful in all cases of chronic disease associated with weakness, poor appetite, and general low energy. It is also helpful in states of emotional depression, helping to lighten the mood. I also like to use oats for treating anxiety, insomnia, irritability, and restlessness. Think of using the herb for both physical and mental fatigue. Oats also have a beneficial action on the heart, strengthening and regulating its function.

The oat grain makes a soothing bath or wash for irritated skin rashes, poison ivy, and itchiness of the skin. The grain is also a nutritious food containing vitamins B1, B2, and E; carotenes; calcium; silica; and proteins. The grass is often added to mineral teas that contain other high mineral plants such as nettles and horsetail.

Preparations and dosages:

Decoction: Use 1 to 2 teaspoons of oat grass to 8 of ounces of water. Cover, simmer for 3 to 5 minutes, and strain. Drink 1 cup, 3 times a day.

Fluid extract or glycerite: Use 1 teaspoon, 3 times a day.

Topical uses: Use a wash with the grain or the grass for healing and soothing the skin. Fill a clean cotton sock or a small linen bag with a cup of oats and put in the bath or use as a body scrub. A few drops of lavender essential oil can be added to the oats for a more relaxing bath.

RED CLOVER *Trifolium pratense*

Part used: Flower

Actions: Alterative, antispasmodic, expectorant, dermatological agent

Uses:

The beautiful red-purple clover is a common meadow flower that makes a delightful tea when mixed with herbs like lemon balm, spearmint, chamomile, and nettles. Its healing action on the skin and its supportive action on the body's immune and eliminatory systems make it especially useful in eczema, psoriasis, acne, and rashes of various types. It is best used over a period of six to twelve months for these conditions. Making a tea or placing 30 drops of tincture in 2 ounces of warm water makes excellent gargling options for treating inflamed sore throats and glands. The herb may also be used for coughs and colds; it aids in reducing the spasm of a cough as well as clearing out mucus. I find the herb most beneficial when a child is weak or has a chronic illness and needs to regain body strength.

Preparations and dosages:

Infusion: Use 2 to 3 teaspoons to 8 ounces of boiling water. Steep for 3 to 5 minutes and strain. Give 1 to 3 cups a day, in ½ to 1 cup doses.

Tincture or glycerite: Use ½ to 1 teaspoon, 3 times a day.

Topical uses: Use for skin rash, bites, stings, or burns. Baths, footbaths, and gargles can all be made from a strong infusion of the herb. Use a quart of tea added to the bath. This can be used for fungal infections of the skin, athlete's foot, or sore throat.

RED RASPBERRY *Rubus idaeus*

Parts used: Leaves and berries

Actions: Astringent, antidiarrheal, uterine tonic

Uses:

The raspberry plant is well-known for its delicious red berries used in desserts, yet few are aware of its medicinal value. The fruit can be used in the form of a vinegar or syrup for loose stools or diarrhea, but the leaf is the more commonly used medicinal part, relieving nausea and vomiting and relaxing the tummy. A strong tea made from the leaves given in tablespoon doses every 15 minutes will slow diarrhea. The plant is astringent in action and can relieve irritation and inflammation in the bowels. A wash of well-strained tea can be used for inflamed eyes, mouth, throat, or skin. Raspberry leaves make a pleasant-tasting tea that blends easily with other herbs served in a hot or cold tea or in an herbal popsicle. The leaves also have a toning effect on the female reproductive system.

Preparations and dosages:

Infusion: Use 1 teaspoon to 8 ounces of boiling water. Steep for 3 to 5 minutes and strain. Give 1 to 3 cups a day, in ½ to 1 cup doses.

Tincture or glycerite: Use ½ to 1 teaspoon, 3 times a day.

Vinegar

Place 1 cup fresh raspberries in a clean jar. Cover with white distilled vinegar so that no berries are uncovered. Let steep for 5 to 7 days and strain. This makes an excellent salad vinegar or a diarrhea remedy, given at ½ teaspoon in ¼ cup of warm water and sipped slowly 2 to 3 times a day.

Syrup of the Fruit

Use 2 cups fresh raspberries to ½ cup vegetable glycerine or raw sugar. Puree the berries and simmer uncovered for 20 minutes, stirring often. Strain out the seeds and put the strained juice back into the pot with the sweetener, and simmer gently for 20 minutes. Cool and bottle. Use 1 to 3 teaspoons, 3 times a day.

ROSEMARY   *Rosmarinus officinalis*

Part used: Leaves

Actions: Antimicrobial, antispasmodic, carminative, vasodilation of the small vessels

Uses:
Rosemary is an aromatic, culinary herb that also has medicinal qualities. The wonderful scent is soothing and calming to the body, making it useful in reducing tension and stress. It is said to be strengthening to the memory and mind. One of the actions of the herb is to increase circulation to the head, hands, and feet, thereby increasing the amount of oxygen that reaches the brain. Because it also increases the flow of blood to the hands and feet, rosemary is at the same time helpful in treating chills, colds, and conditions associated with poor circulation.

The volatile oil of the plant also has a calming effect on the tummy, relieving nausea, vomiting, colic, gas, or upset due to nervous tension. The volatile oil also has an antimicrobial action, making it useful in infections of the digestive and respiratory tracts. Thus, rosemary leaf tea can be used as a gargle for sore throats, a tea for a dry cough, or a wash for cuts, stings, and bites. A hot cup of tea sweetened with honey and lemon is excellent for fevers, influenza, or cough.

Rosemary may also be used as a hair rinse, particularly for dark shades of hair. Regular use will ensure healthy hair and scalp. A few drops of the essential oil of the plant can be rubbed on the hairbrush or comb to add shine and prevent head lice. The essential oil can also be added to a bath to relax the body and invigorate the mind, or it can be added to creams and ointments as an antiseptic.

Preparations and dosages:

Infusion: Use 1 teaspoon to 8 ounces of water. Steep covered, for 3 to 5 minutes. Use 1 to 3 cups a day, in 1-teaspoon to ½-cup doses, 3 to 4 times a day.

Tincture or glycerite: Use ¼ to ½ teaspoon, 3 times a day.

Topical uses: Compresses and skin washes made from strong infusions of rosemary make excellent antiseptic applications and aid in healing the skin from cuts, bites, and stings. Oils and creams of rosemary can be used for their antiseptic qualities, to relax the muscles and increase circulation to the area. Rosemary massage oil can be stimulating to the circulation while relaxing the muscles and encouraging the lymphatic flow.

SAGE *Salvia officinalis*

Part used: Leaves

Actions: Antimicrobial, antiseptic, antispasmodic, astringent, carminative, reduces secretions such as saliva, lactation, and sweat.

Uses:

This culinary herb has a special affinity for the mouth, tongue, and throat. As a gargle, it is useful in healing inflammations of the gums, mouth, tongue, and throat. It dries up excessive secretions of the mouth and throat, reducing phlegm or mucus. Sage tea makes an excellent gargle for sore throats, reducing the irritation and acting as an antiseptic. It has these same effects when applied topically to the skin, making it useful for skin irritations, cuts, and sores. I also like to use it as a wash, footbath, or cream for fungal infections of the skin. Sage tea will settle an upset stomach, reduce gas and bloating, and improve digestive functioning overall. The tea may also be useful to breast-feeding mothers who are weaning their infants, as it will help to dry up the breast milk. Externally, the tea may be used as a hair rinse for treating dandruff or sores of the scalp or for darkening the hair. Use as the final rinse and do not wash out.

Preparations and dosages:

Infusion: Use ½ to 1 teaspoon to 8 ounces of boiling water. Steep for 1 to 3 minutes and strain. Use ¼ to ½ cup, 3 times a day. Use a strong infusion, 2 to 4 times a day, as a gargle.

Tincture or glycerite: Use ¼ to ½ teaspoon, 3 times a day.

Topical uses: Baths, skin washes, or compresses made from a strong infusion of sage can be used to encourage wound healing, avoid infection, and decrease swelling. Creams and salves made of sage are antibacterial and antifungal. They are excellent for diaper rash, athlete's foot, candida rash, or ringworm. Apply several times a day.

SIBERIAN GINSENG *Eleutherococcus senticosus*

Part used: Root

Actions: Adaptogen, immunomodulator, and tonic

Uses:

Like ashwagandha, this herb has a traditional use as a tonic for improving health and stamina, also having a beneficial effect on the growth of muscle tissue in children. I like to mix the two herbs together in a formula for children under stress who have low growth rates or have had a serious illness. This plant has been the topic of much research because of its action as an adaptogen. It acts to assist the body in counteracting and adapting to all types of stress, acting to restore and improve the body's immune response and increasing vitality. It affects mental performance, improving concentration and alertness as well as affecting physical performance, stamina, and the body's ability to withstand adverse conditions, such as heat. This plant can be used in the treatment of hyperactivity, ADD, and ADHD. Remember to include it in formula for use during convalescence periods following antibiotic treatments, acute fever higher than 102°F, severe acute disease, or after surgery.

Preparations and dosages:
Decoction: Use as a tea, 1 to 3 times a day, for several weeks. Most children will prefer it to be sweetened or mixed with more pleasant-tasting herbs such as fennel seed, licorice root, cinnamon bark, peppermint, or stevia.

Tincture: Use ¼ to ½ teaspoon, 1 to 3 times a day, of a 1 to 5 strength extract.

Glycerite: Use ½ to 1 teaspoon, 1 to 3 times a day.

Solid extract: This is a concentrated extract, which has a pastelike consistency and contains no alcohol. It is several times stronger than a tincture or glycerite. A dose of ⅛ to ¼ teaspoon is added to warm water, tea, or juice. The extract can be used morning and evening. Gaia Herbs makes this product.

SKULLCAP *Scutellaria laterifolia*

Part used: Whole herb

Actions: Antispasmodic, mild sedative, tonic for nervous system, relaxant

Uses:
Skullcap has appreciable sedative effects, but it is more noted for its effect as a tonic and builder of the nervous system. This makes skullcap applicable for seizures and hysterical states. It is also indicated for exhausted and depressive states, where the nervous

system has been under prolonged stress or anxiety. It is particularly useful for nervous excitement and restlessness in overtired children or for children who are hyperactive. Skullcap is also effective for nervous disorders characterized by irregular muscle action such as tremors, twitching, and restlessness with or without lack of coordination. Its action continues for a time even after treatment has stopped. Its effects are cumulative so it is most useful if given regularly over a prolonged time rather than in one or two isolated doses.

Skullcap can be mixed with hops and chamomile for sleeplessness, with passionflower for hyperactivity, or with catnip for stomach cramps. It makes a lovely addition to calming herbal baths or sleep pillows.

Preparations and dosages:

Infusion: Use 1 teaspoon to 8 ounces of boiling water. Steep for 3 to 5 minutes and strain. Give 1 to 3 cups a day, in ½- to 1-cup doses, or add to the bath for sleepless, overactive children or to treat muscle aches and pains.

Tincture or glycerite: Use ½ to 1 teaspoon, 3 times a day.

SLIPPERY ELM *Ulmus fulva*

Part used: Inner bark

Actions: Anti-inflammatory, demulcent, emollient, nutrient, vulnerary

Uses:

Many of slippery elm's uses stem from its demulcent or emollient actions, coming from the mucilage in the plant. It is essential to relieve a burning, hot tummy; to quiet diarrhea; or to soothe the itch of diaper rash. Internally, the powder, made into a tea or gruel, will be useful in quieting nausea and vomiting when given in teaspoon doses every 10 minutes. The same tea or gruel is useful with diarrhea or hemorrhoids. The plant decreases irritations to the membranes that line the respiratory passages, making it useful for dry, irritated coughs; sore throats; and ulcers of the mouth. I think of it for any hot, irritated state of the membranes of the nose, throat, lungs, stomach, bowels, or skin.

The inner bark of the slippery elm tree is high in minerals, making it a nutritive herb that is excellent for treating children in feeble, debilitated states. I suggest mixing it with a little cinnamon powder and maple syrup.

For external use on the skin, I like it best as a powder or poultice. The powder can be mixed with other herbs that are healing to the skin such as calendula, comfrey, or lavender and then used to treat all types of rashes, dry up weepy wounds, or protect the skin. The poultice is useful for its drawing properties, making it helpful in drawing a splinter or the sting from a bug bite to the surface or in easing the tenderness of a boil.

Preparations and dosages:

Infusion: Use 1 teaspoon powder to 6 to 8 ounces of boiling
  water. Stir while adding the water to help mix the powder
  smoothly. The tea has a slippery feeling and can be made
  thick or thin, depending on the amount of water used. Give
  ½ to 1 cup, 3 times a day.

Topical uses: Use as a skin powder for diaper rash, weepy
  eczema, fungal infections, or as a foot powder. (See Recipes
  and Remedies for Infants and Children, starting on page
  265.) The gruel can also be used topically for splinters,
  boils, bug bites, cuts, and burns.

Gruel

Use 1 teaspoon powder to 3 tablespoons of boiling water and mix into a paste. If the paste is too thick, add a little more water to thin to desired consistency. Use 1 to 2 teaspoons per dose, 3 to 4 times a day.

ST. JOHN'S WORT *Hypericum perforatum*

Parts used: Whole herb and flowers

Actions: Antiviral, astringent, analgesic, antiseptic, anti-depressant, anti-inflammatory, sedative, restorative to the nervous system

Uses:

I first learned to use this herb as an oil, which is helpful in treating nerve pain such as sciatica or neuralgia. The oil, which is red, also eases the pain of earaches and heals burns and bruises. Internally, the plant has traditionally been used in treating conditions of the nervous system, such as anxiety and overexcitability. Recently, modern researchers have found it to be effective in the treatment of depression. The mood-lightening effect takes several weeks to manifest, and the herb should be taken over several months before assessing its usefulness. Recent research also supports its use as an antiviral, making it helpful in combating chronic viral conditions, stomach viruses, and respiratory virus.

Note: The plant may cause a photosensitive rash in some people. If this occurs, the rash will disappear once the herb has been discontinued.

Preparations and dosages:

Infusion: Use 1 teaspoon to 8 ounces of boiling water. Steep for
5 minutes and strain. Give ½ to 1 cup, 3 times a day. Add
to the bath for nerve pain, muscle pain, overexcitability, or
nervousness.

Tincture or glycerite: Use ¼ to ½ teaspoon, 3 times a day.

Topical uses: Use for earaches, nerve pain, burns, or sores.

THYME *Thymus vulgaris*

Part used: Whole herb

Actions: Antiseptic, antiviral, antibacterial, astringent, expectorant, spasmolytic, urinary antiseptic

Uses:

This aromatic culinary herb is one of my favorite herbal remedies for respiratory infections, such as bronchitis and pneumonia. It is useful in all cough treatments, as it breaks up congestion, warms the mucous membranes, and aids in expelling catarrh. The volatile oil of thyme is highly antimicrobial and is excreted from the body through the lungs and urinary tract, making the remedy particularly useful for infections in those body systems. It can also be added to asthma remedies for its action in breaking up thick secretions and for its relaxing action on the respiratory muscles. Like most of the other aromatic herbs, thyme has a calming effect on the stomach, aiding digestion and relieving gas and bloating. A tea given in teaspoon doses every 15 minutes may be helpful in slowing diarrhea. Use as a gargle made from a tea or add 30 drops of tincture to 2 ounces of warm water for tonsillitis, laryngitis, or general sore throat.

Topically, it can be used in creams or salves for skin fungus, as an herbal oil for fungal ear infections such as swimmer's ear, or as an antiseptic wash for cuts and abrasions. Thyme was also used in folk medicine as a worm remedy.

Preparations and dosages:

Infusion: Use 1 teaspoon to 8 ounces of boiling water. Cover, steep for 1 to 3 minutes, and strain. Use 1 to 3 cups a day, in ¼- to ½-cup doses.

Tincture or glycerite: Use ½ to 1 teaspoon, 3 times a day.

Topical uses: Also can be used in baths, creams, salves, ear oil, or skin washes.

Syrup of the flowering tops: Use 1 teaspoon, 3 times a day.

WILLOW   *Salix alba* and spp.

Part used: Bark

Actions: Analgesic, anti-inflammatory, antipyretic, astringent

Uses:
There are several kinds of willows that are used medicinally for their pain-relieving action. The bark contains a substance that the body turns into salicylic acid. The most common form used today is acetylsalicylic acid, better known as aspirin. The effects of willow bark are the same as aspirin but to a lesser degree. Thus, willow, often called "nature's aspirin," can be used to treat headaches, fevers, and all types of body pain. It has long been used in herbal medicine for arthritic pain, gout, and toothache. I like to use it with wintergreen or meadowsweet for headaches and pain.

Preparations and dosages:
Decoction: Use 1 to 2 teaspoons to 8 ounces of water. Gently simmer for 10 minutes and strain. Give 1 to 3 cups a day, in ½- to 1-cup doses.
Tincture or glycerite: Use ½ teaspoon, 3 times a day.
Topical uses: Use as an herbal oil for painful joints or muscles or for swelling. Make a strong decoction and use as a fomentation.

WINTERGREEN *Gaultheria procumbens*

Part used: Leaves

Actions: Anti-inflammatory, analgesic, diuretic

Uses:

Wintergreen, also known as teaberry or checkerberry, is a common woodland plant found in the northeastern part of the United States. As a child I remember gathering and chewing wintergreen leaves to taste the wonderfully sweet flavor. The plant contains salicylates that act as an anti-inflammatory, thus reducing pain. Like willow, it is often called one of nature's aspirins. Medicinally, it can be used for headaches, muscle aches, and pains and swellings of the joints and muscles. The herb is very pleasant tasting, making it easy to give to children as an addition to any herbal tea blend. Use it topically for a rub or bath when treating headache, sprains, joint pains, or sore muscles.

Preparations and dosages:

Infusion: Use 1 to 2 teaspoons of the dry herb to 8 ounces of boiling water. Steep for 3 to 5 minutes and strain. Use 1 to 3 cups a day, in ½- to 1-cup doses.

Tincture or glycerite: Use ¼ to ½ teaspoon, 3 times a day.

Topical uses: Use 1 tablespoon to 1 pint boiling water. Simmer for 3 to 5 minutes covered. Strain and add to bath water. Use as an herbal oil over swollen or sore area, several times a day.

YARROW *Achillea millefolium*

Parts used: Flowers mainly, but the whole herb can be used

Actions: Astringent, antipyretic, anti-inflammatory, antispasmodic, bitter tonic, diaphoretic, peripheral vasodilator, hypotensive, refrigerant, styptic

Uses:

Yarrow is a common wildflower found in meadows and along roadsides. It has a long history of medicinal use, ranging from treatment of fevers to toothaches. It is both an anti-inflammatory and a refrigerant due to its volatile oils. This makes it very useful when treating fevers, colds and flus, swollen glands, and swellings in general. Its diaphoretic properties also aid in the treatment of fever, increasing sweat. For a fever, yarrow may be used as a hot tea or bath. One of my favorite teas for fevers, colds, and flus is a mixture of yarrow, elder flowers, and peppermint. Yarrow acts on the gastrointestinal tract as a carminative, an antispasmodic, and as a mild bitter. These qualities make the herb particularly useful in influenza and respiratory infections associated with fever, malaise, and decreased appetite. One of its beneficial effects when taken over time is to tonify the digestive system, making it stronger. Yarrow can be very useful with children who have chronic stomachaches, gas, bloating, and poor stool habits.

Yarrow also increases blood flow to the hands and feet, thus aiding poor circulation and bringing a warming sensation to the skin. This herb also acts locally in external topical applications as a compress, bath, or cream used to decrease inflammation and promote healing of the skin as well as to stop bleeding.

Preparations and dosages:

Infusion: Use 1 teaspoon of the dry herb to 8 ounces of boiling
water. Steep for 1 to 2 minutes and strain. Sweeten with

honey, as the tea can be bitter. Give 1 to 3 cups a day, in teaspoon to ½-cup doses.

Tincture or glycerite: Use ¼ to ½ teaspoon, 3 times a day.

Topical uses: Use 1 tablespoon to 1 pint of boiling water. Steep 10 to 20 minutes and strain into the bath. Use as a cream or ointment on the skin to decrease inflammation and promote healing.

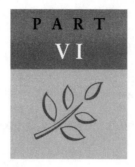

The Herbal Pharmacy

THE CHEMISTRY OF PLANTS

Plants have been sources of medicines for generations. Many modern pharmaceutical medicines are based on plant-derived substances, and plant compounds are continually being studied for their possible medicinal value in the modern world. The chemical compounds of many plants are being isolated and used in the production of phytomedicines or manufactured synthetically and used in the production of pharmaceutical medicines. The pharmaceutical approach, which reduces a medicinal herb to that of its chemical components, is rather limiting because the chief active components of the herb are of primary importance yet are only a part of the whole. Many secondary chemical compounds support the chief compound, buffer harsh side effects, or enhance the body's receptiveness to the herb. Herbalists feel it is most valuable to use the whole herb in medicinal applications, getting the full benefit of all its compounds. The whole plant offers more of nature's safeguards. Overall, the whole plant is far safer and gentler than its isolated compounds.

Active Chemical Compounds

The following are found in plants and are known to have specific therapeutic actions in the body.

Alkaloids

These organic nitrogen compounds usually appear in groups. They are very potent plant compounds that relieve pain and sedate the central nervous system, but they are often toxic in large amounts. For these reasons, many medicinal herbs high in alkaloids should be used only by trained herbal practitioners. A few commonly known alkaloids include caffeine found in coffee, cocoa, and black tea and nicotine found in tobacco, both of which have strong effects on the central nervous system. Alkaloids are also found in the following herbs: ephedra, lobelia, comfrey, and coltsfoot.

Bitters

This compound includes a number of different chemical groups such as glycosides, alkaloids, and resins. These kinds of plants have a bitter taste and a direct action on the digestive tract, beginning in the mouth. They promote secretion of saliva, hydrochloric acid, and digestive enzymes in the stomach, small intestines, and pancreas and bile in the liver. At the same time, they increase stomach and intestinal movement and stabilize blood sugar. Bitters are used to tone up sluggish digestion, increase the appetite, and promote good bowel movements.

Other uses for bitter herbs include relieving liver congestion, gastritis, anemia, allergies, and skin conditions. One of the keys to ensuring the effectiveness of a bitter herb on the digestive tract is to take it by mouth and experience its bitter taste. A common way to administer bitters is to add 30 drops to 2 ounces of water and sip ½ hour before meals, 1 to 3 times a day. Bitter herbs include gentian, dandelion, peppermint, and hops.

Flavonoids

This glycoside (see next section) is responsible for the red, yellow, or orange color of flowers, fruits, and vegetables. They act as antioxidants, decreasing free radical damage in the body. Flavonoids improve the strength and durability of the blood vessels. They are useful in all types of cardiovascular disease. Flavonoids also stabilize inflammation in the body, making them useful in the treatment of allergies, eczema, colds, and infections. They increase vitamin C utilization in the cells. Herbs high in flavonoids include hawthorne berry, bilberry, and black currant.

Glycosides

Glycosides are two-sectioned molecules made up of sugar and nonsugar components. They yield one or more sugars upon hydrolysis at the active site. Glycosides contribute to almost every therapeutic class of herbs and are found widely in the plant world. A special group of glycosides known as the cardiac glycosides have a special effect on the heart muscle and its rhythm. These plants are used for the treatment of heart failure, arrhythmias, weak heart, and for stabilizing the function of the heart muscle. Herbs in this group include wild oats and lily of the valley.

Mucilages

These gelatinous substances are made up of proteins and poly-saccharides (sugars). They are very soothing to inflamed tissue and are used for their demulcent and emollient properties. When the dry herb or powder is mixed with water, it forms a viscous, gel-like substance which, when taken into the bowel, will cause a bulking effect, pulling water into the bowel and causing a mild laxative action. Flax and psyllium seed are used for this action. Mucilages also absorb excessive lung secretions, decreasing catarrh, while soothing bronchial irritations and inflammations. Thus, they are useful in cough syrups and teas, as with slippery elm and marshmallow root. Used to relieve stomachaches, heartburn, and ulcers of the digestive tract, they decrease irritation and burning and promote healing of the tissue. They have a general softening action on the tissues that they come into contact with, internally and externally.

Saponins

This type of glycoside creates a soapy lather when mixed with water. Overall, they are not well-absorbed by the digestive tract but help to promote digestion and absorption of other substances such as minerals. They irritate the membranes of the lungs thereby producing a watery secretion and a cough, which then moves the mucus out of the lungs. Some act as diuretics by irritating the urinary mucous membranes and increasing the amount of fluid excreted through the kidneys. Some saponins have steroidal structures similar to those of human hormones. These steroidal saponin plants can regulate hormonal activity in the body, counter the effects of stress, and decrease inflammation through their anti-inflammatory action. Plants known to contain large amounts of steroidal saponins include Siberian ginseng, wild yam, licorice, and fenugreek.

Tannins

These common plant constituents are responsible for the astringent action of medicinal plants. They bind proteins, alkaloids, and gelatin. This causes a tight protective barrier that is resistant to microbes, inflammation, and irritants. Thus, they decrease irritation, inflammation, and infection in the membranes lining the nose, throat, lungs, eyes, digestive system, urinary system, and skin. They will aid in healing wounds, burns, and rashes when used in skin washes, baths, or salves. They are common additions to gargles and mouthwashes for sore throats, swollen glands, and gum infections or bleeding. They are useful in treating diarrhea because they reduce irritation and decrease the loss of fluid from the intestines. Use high-tannin plants as compresses for hemorrhoids, swellings, or abrasions. Some herbs that are high in tannins include witch hazel, raspberry, white oak bark, and bayberry root.

Volatile Oils

Volatile oils are complex plant compounds that are made up of hydrocarbons and alcohols. In the plant, they often enhance the moisture-retaining properties of the leaves. They give taste and fragrance to herbs, as in rosemary, lavender, thyme, mint, and anise. They act as antiseptics, antifungals, and antimicrobials. This makes them useful in helping the immune system fight off infections. Many volatile oils are anti-inflammatory, such as wintergreen, chamomile, and yarrow, and help to reduce skin and muscle inflammation. Some oils like thyme or eucalyptus stimulate the release of mucus from the lungs via their expectorant action if used as a steam or inhalant. Topically, volatile oils stimulate the skin when used in a massage oil or friction rub. They relax the muscles bringing warmth and increasing lymphatic and blood flow. Volatile oils are active in the digestive tract when ingested through food, teas, extracts, or tablets. They are excreted from the body through the urinary system, the respiratory system, and through body secretions such as sweat, saliva, breast milk, and tears. Thus, the oils have an effect on these systems, too. Many of the volatile oils are used in the ancient healing art of aromatherapy for their actions on the emotional body. These oils stimulate the olfactory nerves that carry impulses to the brain, particularly to the limbic center, which governs emotional states of being. Oils like rose, lavender, chamomile, lemon balm, and peppermint are often used in this way as baths, massage oils, or perfumes.

HARVESTING, DRYING, AND STORING HERBS

Learning how to harvest, dry, and store medicinal and culinary herbs can be fun and exciting. It can give you the opportunity to grow some of your own medicines and health-supportive teas. It opens up a world of new healing agents among these plants with their wondrous smells, tastes, and influences on your body. Working with the plants in this way will widen your relationship with them and your knowledge of their applications.

When harvesting herbs, be sure to collect plants that are not rotting, soiled, eaten by bugs, or overripe. You'll want fresh, healthy herbs when collecting for medicinal use. Gather the herbs in unpolluted areas and away from roadsides and power lines. Do not let fresh herbs overheat in the collecting containers, as that will start the process of decomposition and cause the loss of therapeutic compounds. When gathering in the wild, be careful not to overpick in any one area, and spread some seed to encourage regrowth.

Harvesting Plant Parts

Bark is best harvested in the early spring when the sap is rising or in the autumn when the sap is about to fall. Look for the last yellow leaf. Dry whole, or cut into one-inch strips. Examples: Crampbark, wild cherry, willow.

Flowers are best when picked on a warm dry day after the dew has evaporated and the flowers are fully mature and still robust—when the bees like them. The flowers will often pop off easily when ripe. Dry them by spreading them out on a screen. Examples: Calendula, chamomile.

Leaves are best when harvested on a warm day just after the dew has dried off the plant in the morning, just before flowering, or when setting buds. Whole stems are usually collected and stripped off after drying. Examples: Mints, lemon balm, nettles.

Roots or rhizomes have varying harvest times. If the plant is a biennial, harvest the root in the autumn of the first year or spring of the second year before a lot of foliage growth has occurred, as with burdock. If it is a perennial plant, harvest in the autumn before the first deep frost and after the tops have died back or in the very early spring before foliage activity. Wash and chop into one-half-inch pieces before drying. Examples: Comfrey, elecampane.

Whole herbs consist of all aerial parts of the plant such as the leaves, flowers, and stems. Harvest on a warm day in the morning after the dew has dried, just when the flowers are starting to bloom and are heavy with buds. Dry on the stem in small bundles. Examples: Catnip, hyssop.

Seeds or fruits should be harvested when fully grown, just as they ripen. Example: Hawthorne.

Drying

Plants contain a large amount of water. Roots usually dry to approximately one-half their fresh weight and leaves to one-eighth to one-tenth of their fresh weight. One must remove sufficient moisture to prevent molding, bacterial contamination, or enzymatic or chemical changes. Some changes that occur in the drying process are desirable, as they provide a last chemical change for the production of active constituents, such as with gentian or wild cherry. Direct sunlight generally depletes the physical and chemical properties of plants. It is used to dry some roots (those containing tannins and anthraquinone glycosides), but as a general rule it is not advisable to dry herbs in the sun. Proper circulation of air is essential for good drying. Choose a well-ventilated room for drying. Use a fan to ensure good air circulation and prevent mold from growing.

Take caution not to overdry. The active ingredients can be affected and the results will be inferior. Leaves and flowers should be dry but not crumbly or excessively brittle.

Storage Instructions

When deciding where to store your herbs, consider the following:

- Air facilitates oxidation, so fill containers to the top with the herb, or fill the excess space with cotton.
- Light causes photo-oxidation and accelerates chemical changes in the herb. Polarized light is worse than ordinary light, and all reflected light is polarized to some extent. Thus, it is essential to use opaque containers or to store clear glass jars in a closed cabinet or closet.

- Temperature affects the rate of chemical reaction in plant material. The higher the temperature, the more the rate of chemical reaction increases. Ideal storage temperature is 55°F to 65°F.
- Remove all insects, fungus, material, bacteria, and other contaminants before putting into storage containers.
- To avoid having to open the jars frequently, have a stock container to store large amounts of the herb and smaller ones for regular use that can be filled from the stock container.

Storage Containers

Airtight glass containers are best. Avoid plastic, as it can be broken down by some of the active constituents in the herbs. Hard plastic containers are okay for short-term use, but glass is best. Make sure to protect the herb matter from light. Use amber jars or keep clear glass jars in an herb closet to shut out the light. The atmosphere should be dry. Before filling, all containers should be heated slightly to eliminate condensation, then cooled and the herb matter put inside immediately. If there is any extra moisture in the jar, the herb will mold. Enzymes stay active in the plant matter at 8- to 10-percent moisture content and cause deterioration.

Most dried leaves and flowers can be kept up to a year and replenished with a new harvest each growing season. Roots, barks, and seeds will store longer, as they consist of harder plant materials; they should keep eighteen to thirty-six months.

MAKING HERBAL PREPARATIONS

Many herbal preparations are easy to make at home. Making your own teas, decoctions, oils, salves, and extracts can be simple and lots of fun. Many herbal cosmetic preparations can also be made easily. See recipes at the end of this section.

For making most home herbal preparations, you'll need a minimal amount of equipment. Pots should be stainless steel or glass. Use wooden spoons and avoid aluminum utensils. Here is a list of the basic equipment you will need:

Medium stainless steel or glass pot with cover
Double boiler, glass or stainless steel
Slow cooker, such as a Crock-Pot
Wooden spoons
Cheesecloth
Ladle
Strainers, fine and coarse
Clean Ball jars, quart size
Blender or food processor
Coffee filters
Coffee grinder

Baths

Use a quart of an infusion or a decoction depending on the herb. Strain the herbs out and add the decoction to the bath.

Capsules

Empty gelatin capsules can be purchased at many health food stores or herb shops and then filled with herbal powder. Most capsules are available in size o or oo, the oo being the larger. Most children are better with o size. Dried leaves, flowers, roots, and barks can be powdered in a coffee grinder, sifted through a fine sieve several times, and put into the capsules. Many herb shops carry a selection of herbal powders that can be used in capsules. Remember that herbal powders lose their potency in 12 months, so make sure your source is fresh.

Decoctions

Decoctions are used for the hard or woody parts of the plant, such as the roots, seeds, and barks. The proportions are the same as for an infusion, 1 teaspoon per cup. Place the herb in the cold water, bring to a boil, simmer 5 to 20 minutes, remove from the heat, and strain. Use within 8 to 12 hours or store in the refrigerator for up to 3 days.

Fomentations

These are compresses soaked in an herbal infusion or decoction and applied externally. Make up a quart of an infusion or decoction and use a flannel cloth or washcloth as the compress. Moisten the cloth with the herbal mixture and apply over the affected area. Cover with a piece of plastic and then a towel to keep the compress warm. Leave on for 15 to 25 minutes.

Glycerites

Herbs can be extracted into glycerine by letting the herb digest into it for 10 days. There is a higher risk of mold occurring, as the glycerine is high in sugars, so be sure all the plant matter is covered with glycerine and none is exposed to the air. I prefer to use fresh herbs chopped into small pieces. Put the chopped herb into a clean jar and cover completely with a mixture of 75-percent U.S.P. vegetable glycerine and 25-percent water. Mix the glycerine and water together before pouring over the herbs. Place in a dark, cool place and shake every few days. After 10 days, press out the herb material and bottle.

Infusions

Infusions are made from the aerial parts of the plant, such as leaves and flowers, and sometimes soft berries and seeds. The standard proportion is 1 teaspoon herb to 1 cup of water. Pour the boiling water over the herb, cover, and let stand for 10 to 30 minutes. Most infusions should be used within 8 to 12 hours or can be stored in the refrigerator up to 3 days.

Oils

Herbal oils can be made either by heating or by a no-cook method. The cooking method is quicker. Oils to use include olive, sweet almond, safflower, sesame, or avocado.

Herbal Oil (no-cook method)
All herbs should be chopped or ground (if dried). Put herbs into clear glass jar. Cover with enough oil to completely submerge the herbs. Let sit in a warm sunny place for 10 to 14 days. Strain and bottle. Store in a cool place.

Herbal Oil (cook method)
Prepare herbs and cover with adequate oil. Let cook in low oven 100°F to 150°F for 12 to 15 hours, or use a slow cooker, such as a Crock-Pot, for 12 hours. Strain and bottle. Store in a cool place.

Ointments and Salves

Salves are very simple to make once you have prepared the herbal oil. Often, I will make all of the herbal oils that I want for the season during the summer when the herbs are fresh. Then I use them to make salves later in the year.

General Guidelines

Be sure to follow these guidelines when making ointments or salves.

- Use 2 ounces of beeswax to 1 pint of oil for ointments.
- Avoid petroleum bases.
- Mix 10 to 20 drops of essential oils to each pint of salve to improve the scent, to help penetrate the skin, and to add medicinal qualities.
- Store in tightly closed containers in a cool, dark place. Refrigeration is ideal.
- Use salves and oils within a year for best results.

Directions

Grate beeswax while gently heating the prepared herb oil in a double boiler. Add the grated beeswax and melt. When the beeswax has melted, pour or ladle the hot mixture into small 1-ounce containers before it hardens. If adding essential oils, do it when the mixture has just been taken off the heat.

Poultices

Poultices can be made simply by macerating a fresh herb to a pulp and applying the pulp to the skin. The herb can be crushed by using a mortar and pestle, a blender, or by finely chopping it with a knife. Dried herbs can be used if reconstituted with water until moist and soft. Fresh roots can be grated and applied to the skin as a poultice. Herbal powder can be used for poultices if they are mixed with enough warm water to make a paste or gruel and then applied to the affected area.

Powders (Body)

Dried leaves, flowers, roots, and barks can be powdered in a coffee grinder or sifted through a fine sieve several times. These powders can be put into a shaker or applied with a powder puff.

Many herb shops carry a selection of herbal powders that can be used on the body.

Steams

Herbal steams can be made with either the herb or its volatile oil. When using a volatile oil, use 5 to 8 drops of oil in a large bowl of steaming water. When using an herb, add 1 to 2 tablespoons to a quart of boiling water. Use a towel to create a tent over the bowl and have the child breathe the steam for 3 to 5 minutes.

Syrups

Syrups can be easily made up and stored in the refrigerator for several months. A syrup base can be made by dissolving 2½ pounds of raw sugar in 1 pint of water over a gentle heat. When all the sugar has dissolved, cook for 1 minute and remove from heat. The base syrup can then be mixed with a tincture to make a medicated syrup. Use 1 part tincture to 3 parts syrup.

To make an herbal syrup, start with a pint of an infusion or decoction, and add 1 cup of raw sugar to it. Bring the whole mixture to a boil, remove from heat, cool, and bottle. If you wish to use honey, use equal parts honey and infusion or decoction, and heat slowly to a simmer. Continue simmering until thick, remove from heat, and bottle. Syrups made without using tinctures are best stored in the refrigerator; those with tinctures added can be stored at room temperature.

Tinctures

Tinctures are made by digesting herbs in an alcohol/water mixture for 14 days. They can be made with either fresh or dried herbs, and they provide a way to preserve the medicinal properties for a long time. Officially, a tincture contains 1 part herb to 5 parts 100-percent alcohol/water mixture by weight. A simple home method is to pack a jar with the herb and cover with an alcohol/water solution so that no herb matter is exposed to the air. Let stand for 14 days. Press or strain out the herb and bottle in amber bottles. It is best to use 100-percent grain alcohol, but a good-quality vodka will work for the home method. When using vodka use a 50-percent proof, and no dilution with water will be necessary. When using 100-percent grain alcohol dilute to desired strength. A 50-percent alcohol/50-percent water mixture will extract most medicinal constituents from common medicinal herbs.

RECIPES AND REMEDIES FOR INFANTS AND CHILDREN

Fresh Glycerite of Lance Leaf Plantain or Ribwort
This makes a cough syrup base to add to other lung tinctures; or add ½ teaspoon to an herbal lung tea. The ribwort dries the membranes if they are producing excessive amounts of mucus and soothes irritations of the membranes. Lance leaf plantain is preferred over broadleaf plantain as a lung herb.

1 lb. fresh ribwort leaves
Vegetable glycerine

Either juice the ribwort leaves or add a small amount of water and puree in the blender. Strain. Add 50-percent glycerine. Store in the refrigerator. Other herbs that can be prepared this way include cleavers, nettles, and dandelion leaf.

Onion Cough Syrup
This makes a wonderful base for adding tinctures of other cough and flu herbs such as thyme, elecampane, echinacea,

yarrow, or mullein. Add equal amounts of tinctured herb mix to onion syrup, such as ¼ ounce thyme tincture and ¼ ounce echinacea tincture to ½ ounce onion syrup.

1 medium onion, sliced
1–2 cups raw sugar

Layer sugar and slices of onion in a glass jar until full. Let sit in a cool place for 1 to 2 days. Strain out onion and bottle in an amber jar. Store in refrigerator or in a cool place. Use ½ to 1 teaspoon, 3 times a day.

Syrup of Marshmallow

Excellent for dry cough or sore throat. Herbal tinctures may also be added to the syrup.

2 oz. marshmallow root, sliced or cut
1½ cups sugar
1 cup distilled water

Soak marshmallow root in water for 12 hours. Add sugar and heat to a boil; cool and strain through cheesecloth. Bottle and store in the refrigerator.

Mucilage of Comfrey

This makes an excellent topical gel for burns, wounds, rashes, bug bites, and swellings.

Soak 4 ounces comfrey root in 2 quarts cold water for 12 hours. Heat to a boil, then simmer for 45 to 60 minutes, uncovered. Strain root out.

The mucilage may be preserved with 6 ounces of honey or 4 ounces of glycerine if using internally for coughs, bowel irritations, or inflammations.

Mullein/Lobelia Neck Wrap
for Sore Throats, Tonsillitis, and Laryngitis

1 oz. verbascum leaf
½ oz. lobelia
1 tsp. cayenne
1 pint apple cider vinegar
1 pint water

Put vinegar, water, mullein, and lobelia into a pot, cover, and simmer gently for 15 minutes. Turn off heat and add cayenne. Dip a cloth into the mixture and wrap around the neck. Cover the wrap with plastic and a dry towel to keep the heat in. Change the wrap when cool. Use 1 or 2 times daily, for 10 to 15 minutes, at each application.

Carrot Poultice
This is helpful for sore throats, especially with children. Grate 2 large carrots, spread onto a thin cloth (cheesecloth is best), and fold the cloth so that carrot is enclosed. Wrap around the throat and secure with a safety pin. Cover with an additional scarf or towel. The poultice can be either hot or cold, depending on which feels better. For a cold poultice, combine crushed ice with the carrot. For a hot poultice, place cloth and carrot in hot water and squeeze out before applying to the neck.

Mustard Pack
When placed over the chest, a mustard pack will stimulate the lungs to expectorate or loosen up a tight chest and dry cough. Don't leave on longer than 10 minutes for a child, or 15 to 20 minutes for an adult. Be aware of irritation to the skin. Check every 3 to 5 minutes and remove if skin hurts and is glowing red.

Add 1 to 2 tablespoons dry mustard (depending on its freshness and potency) to 1 cup of flour. Add enough hot water to make a paste. Spread paste over a thin cloth and place another cloth on top, making a mustard sandwich. Apply a light layer of olive oil to chest. Place the cloth over the oiled chest, then 1 layer of plastic wrap with a hot water bottle or heating pad on top.

Castor Oil Pack

This healing aid may be used on any part of the body to decrease inflammation or congestion. Apply when at rest, in a calm, quiet environment. Pack should be in place for 1 to 1½ hours for best results but can be left on for much longer.

Fold 2 to 4 thicknesses of flannel cloth to the appropriate size for the body part. Put cloth on a sheet of plastic wrap and pour castor oil over it, enough to saturate cloth. Apply cloth to skin, cover with plastic wrap, and then a hot water bottle or a heating pad. The saturated flannel cloth may be kept in the refrigerator for future use for up to 2 months.

Chest Rub for Cough and Congestion

Add 20 drops of essential oil (either eucalyptus, hyssop, thyme, peppermint, or basil) to 2 ounces almond or olive oil.

Herbal Inhaler

Fill a 1-ounce bottle with cotton and add 5 to 10 drops of an essential oil. Sniff gently into each nostril several times a day to decongest the nose and sinuses. Oils to choose from include lavender, eucalyptus, peppermint, or rosemary.

Eucalyptus Steam

This acts as an antimicrobial and decongestant for the respiratory tract.

Bring about 1 quart of water to a boil in a nonaluminum pot. Take the pot off stove, add 3 to 5 drops of eucalyptus oil, and quickly drape a towel over the child's head and the pot so the child can inhale the steam. Have the child inhale through the nose and exhale through the mouth for 5 to 10 minutes. This can be done several times daily when acute. Cautions: Be very careful not to burn the face. Never take eucalyptus oil internally.

Skin Powder for Baby's Bottom

2 parts slippery elm powder
1 part lavender flowers, powdered
1 part calendula flowers, powdered

Mix thoroughly and put in a powder shaker. Shake onto baby's bottom.

Skin Powder for Diaper Rash

2 parts slippery elm powder
1 part bentonite clay
1 part calendula flowers, powdered
1 part goldenseal powder

Prepare as in previous recipe.

Umbilical Cord Powder

This powder will help to keep the cord stump dry and free of infection.

Mix together ½ ounce each of slippery elm powder and goldenseal powder. Apply to baby's umbilical cord after applying alcohol and drying 3 or 4 times a day.

Skin Wash for Chicken Pox, Measles, or German Measles
1 oz. burdock root
½ oz. yarrow flowers
½ oz. chickweed or plantain leaves

Add burdock root to 1 quart of cold water and bring to a boil. Simmer 15 minutes and remove from heat. Add yarrow and chickweed or plantain and steep, covered, for 10 minutes. This mixture may be stored in the refrigerator for 3 days and brought to the desired temperature as needed.

Skin Wash for Poison Ivy, Oak, or Hemlock
1 part sassafras root
1 part burdock root
1 part comfrey root
1 part marshmallow root

Add 2 ounces of root mix to 2 pints of cold water. Bring to a boil and simmer 10 minutes, covered, then steep for 10 minutes. Add ½ pint apple cider vinegar. Use as a wash or in a bath.

Basic Ear Oil
Use ½ ounce each of mullein oil, St. John's wort oil, and calendula oil.

Possible additions:

- Garlic oil or goldenseal glycerite for acute bacterial infection

- Ma huang or lobelia for narrowing of the eustachian tube
- Lobelia oil for severe pain
- Plantain glycerite for chronic catarrh and fluid

Lobelia Preparations

Lobelia is a powerful antispasmodic and pain reliever when used topically for stomach pain, gas, colic, constipation, or bowel pain.

Lobelia Oil

Use 4 ounces freshly picked lobelia herb that has been chopped finely or pulverized in 8 to 10 ounces of olive oil. Allow to soak, shaking daily for 7 days. Strain and bottle with 1 400 I.U. vitamin E capsule, the contents of which will preserve the oil.

Lavender and Lobelia Fomentation

Mix 2 teaspoons lavender flowers and 1 teaspoon lobelia herb in a large glass bowl. Cover with 16 ounces of boiling water and steep, covered, for 10 minutes. Soak a cotton or flannel cloth in the infusion and apply to child's stomach at a comfortable temperature. Cover with a towel and leave in place 5 to 15 minutes.

Lavender and Lobelia Oil Pack

Mix 2 ounces of lobelia oil with 20 drops of lavender oil and saturate a cotton or flannel cloth with the mixture. Apply the cloth over the stomach and intestinal area and cover with a hot water bottle or heating pad for 15 minutes.

Creams and Salves

Rosewater Cold Cream
1⅓ oz. almond oil
½ oz. beeswax
1⅓ oz. rose water
10 drops rose essential oil

Coconut Oil Lotion
1⅔ oz. coconut oil
⅔ oz. almond oil
1 oz. orange flower water
20 drops essential oil(s) of choice

The method is the same for cream and lotion recipes. Weigh all ingredients (if using beeswax grate before weighing). Put the beeswax and oil into a double boiler and stir until melted. While oil mixture is heating, gently heat the flower water separately. When the beeswax is melted and the flower water is warm, take them off of the heat and start adding the flower water to the oil mixture a few drops at a time while beating with a whisk. Beat just until all the water has been absorbed and then mix in the essential oils. Put into opaque jars and leave in a cool place to set.

Herbal Burn Salve
Use 2 ounces each of St. John's wort oil, plantain oil, and comfrey oil, following directions for Oils. (See page 262.) Warm the oils in a double boiler, add 1 ounce grated beeswax, and stir gently with a wooden spoon until melted. Cool a minute while stirring. Then add 1 ounce of aloe vera gel. Pour into opaque containers and cool.

Teas

Seed Tea for Colic and Gas

Mix ½ teaspoon each of fennel, anise, and dill seeds in a teapot or glass Ball jar. Add 12 ounces of boiling water, cover, and steep for 10 minutes. For infants, use 1 to 2 droppersful, every ½ hour as needed. For toddlers, use 2 to 3 teaspoons, every ½ hour.

Healthy Herbal Punch for Kids

This makes an excellent warm or cool drink that supports the immune and digestive systems and helps to fight colds, flu, and fever.

Blend ½ ounce of each of the following herbs: chamomile flowers, elder flowers, lemon balm, nettles, red clover, and spearmint.

Pour 2 cups of boiling water over 1 tablespoon of the herbal blend and let steep 5 to 7 minutes. Strain and mix with 2 cups of apple, berry, or grape juice.

Glossary of
Therapeutic Terms

Active constituent. Chemical component of a crude plant that has a therapeutic effect.

Adaptogen. Acts to assist the body in coping with, adapting to, and counteracting the effects of all types of stress on the body.

Adjuvant. Reinforces the effect of another herb. Supports the action of the main herb.

Alterative. Acts to slowly restore the proper function of the body systems and increase health and vitality. Alteratives work to normalize metabolism and increase and support proper elimination.

Analgesic. Relieves pain when given internally.

Anodyne. Relieves pain when applied topically.

Antacid. Counteracts acidity, especially in the stomach. Herbal antacids usually also have demulcent properties for additional protection of the stomach mucosa.

Anthelmintic. Expels or kills worms in the gastrointestinal tract.

Antiasthmatic. Relieves the symptoms of asthma.

Anticatarrhal. Eliminates or counteracts the formation of mucus in the sinus area, lungs, and elsewhere. Anticatarrhals are often combined with herbs that aid in elimination via sweat, urine, and feces.

Antiemetic. Reduces the feeling of nausea; can help relieve or prevent vomiting.

Antilithic. Prevents the formation of calculi of the kidney, gallbladder, or other concentrations in the joints and muscles.

Antipyretic. Counteracts fever and is often sweat-inducing.

Antiseptic. Prevents infection by inhibiting the growth of micro-organisms on living tissue.

Antispasmodic. Eases or prevents skeletal or smooth-muscle spasms.

Antitussive. Inhibits coughs.

Aperient. The mildest form of herbal laxative.

Aromatic. Characterized by a fragrant, pungent, or spicy scent or taste. Stimulates the gastrointestinal mucous membranes. Often used to mask the flavor of unpleasant-tasting herbs.

Astringent. Causes constriction or contraction of the tissues and/or coagulates proteins, thus decreasing fluid discharge from the tissue. Used to stop bleeding, diarrhea, and swelling of the tissues, as in hemorrhoids or glands. This is the main action of most tannins.

Carminative. Expels gas from the stomach and intestines and thus helps to relieve colic and griping; also relaxes the stomach.

Cathartic. A strong laxative used to cleanse the liver, gall ducts, and intestinal canal. Stimulates peristaltic action.

Cholagogue. Acts on the liver, stimulating bile secretion and flow. Stimulates the release of bile from the gallbladder. Promotes the flow of bile into the small intestines.

Choleretic. Stimulates the production of bile.

Counterirritant. Used to produce superficial inflammation of the skin to relieve deeper inflammation, thus allaying deeper pains and restoring function by bringing greater circulation to the area.

Demulcent. A mucilagenous substance taken internally to soothe, soften, and decrease irritation of the mucous membranes.

Depurative. Purifying agents that aid in the elimination of waste.

Diaphoretic. Promotes moderate sweating when used as a hot tea.

Diuretic. Increases the secretion and elimination of urine.

Doctrine of signatures. The theory stating that how a plant looks and grows will reveal its therapeutic value.

Emetic. Induces vomiting.

Emmenagogue. Normalizes menstrual function, promotes menstrual flow; often contraindicated in pregnancy.

Emollient. A mucilagenous substance used externally to soothe, soften, protect, and relieve irritations.

Expectorant. Aids in the expelling of mucus from the lungs and throat.

Febrifuge. Reduces fevers.

Galactagogue. Stimulates milk production and flow.

Hepatic. Tones and strengthens the liver and normalizes the flow of bile.

Hypertensive. Helps to raise low blood pressure.

Immune modulator. Acts to restore, enhance, and improve the body's immune function and response.

Laxative. Stimulates movement of the large colon.

Mucolytic. Breaks up and resolves mucus.

Nervine. Soothes and relieves tension without sedation; may stimulate or relax.

Parturient. Induces or assists labor and in expelling the placenta.

Purgative. Induces copious evacuation of the bowels; used in cleansing and purifying. Not to be used during pregnancy.

Refrigerant. Used to lower body temperature without inducing perspiration.

Rubefacient. Reddens the skin; sometimes used for a superficial counterirritant effect.

Sedative. Decreases central nervous system function, pain, and nervous irritation.

Sialagogue. Induces increased salivation; aids in the digestion of starch.

Soporific. Induces sleep.

Spasmolytic. Decreases spasms. Also called antispasmodic.

Stimulant. Quickens the functional activity of the tissues, produces energy, warms the body, increases circulation, breaks up obstructions.

Stomachic. Stimulates digestion and/or appetite.

Styptic. Stops external bleeding.

Synergistic. The simultaneous action of two or more substances in the plant whose combined effect is greater than the sum of each working part.

Tonic. Improves body tone by stimulating tissue nutrition; invigorates, restores, and stimulates the system; promotes optimal tissue tone.

Trophorestorative. Nourishes a specific system and has a general nourishing effect on the entire body.

Vermicide or vermifuge. Kills or expels intestinal worms.

Vulnerary. Promotes wound healing.

Glossary of Herbs

Common Name	Botanical Name	Part Used
Aloe	*Aloe arboreseens*	Leaves
Anise	*Pimpinella anisum*	Seed
Ashwagandha	*Withania somnifera*	Root
Astragalus	*Astragalus membranaceus*	Root
Bayberry	*Myrica cerifera*	Rootbark
Bilberry	*Vaccinium myrtillus*	Leaves, fruit
Burdock	*Arctium lappa*	Leaves, root, seed
Calendula	*Calendula officinalis*	Flowers
Catnip	*Nepeta cateria*	Whole herb
Celandine	*Chelidonimmajus*	Whole herb
Chamomile	*Matricaria recutita*	Flowers
Cinnamon	*Cinnamomum* spp.	Bark
Cleavers	*Galium aparine*	Whole herb
Comfrey	*Symphytum officinalis*	Leaves, root
Coneflower	*Echinacea* spp.	Root, whole herb

Common Name	Botanical Name	Part Used
Crampbark	*Viburnum opulus*	Bark
Dandelion	*Taraxacum officinale*	Leaves, root
Dill	*Anethum graveolens*	Leaves, seed
Elder	*Sambucus nigra*	Flowers, berries
Elecampane	*Inula helenium*	Root
Eucalyptus	*Eucalyptus* spp.	Leaves
Eyebright	*Euphrasia officinalis*	Whole herb
Fennel	*Foeniculum vulgare*	Seed
Fenugreek	*Trigonella foenum-graecum*	Seed
Garlic	*Allium sativum*	Bulb, cloves
Ginger	*Zingiber officinale*	Root
Ginkgo	*Ginkgo biloba*	Leaves
Goldenseal	*Hydrastis canadensis*	Root
Hawthorne	*Crataegus* spp.	Flowers, berries, leaves
Hops	*Humulus lupulus*	Strobiles
Horse Chestnut	*Aesculus hippocastanum*	Seed
Horsetail	*Equisetum arvense*	Whole herb
Hyssop	*Hyssopus officinalis*	Whole herb
Irish Moss	*Cetraria islandica*	Whole herb
Lavender	*Lavendula officinalis*	Flowers
Lemon Balm	*Melissa officinalis*	Leaves
Lichen	*Usnea barbata*	Herb
Licorice	*Glycyrrhiza glabra*	Root
Linden	*Tillia* spp.	Flowers
Ma Huang	*Ephedra sinica*	Herb
Marshmallow	*Althea officinalis*	Root, leaves
Meadowsweet	*Filipendula ulmaria*	Whole herb
Mullein	*Verbascum thapsus*	Leaves, flowers
Myrrh	*Commiphora molmol*	Resin

Common Name	Botanical Name	Part Used
Nettles	*Urtica dioica*	Leaves
Oats	*Avena sativa*	Whole herb, seeds
Osha	*Ligusticum porteri*	Root
Parsley	*Petroselinum crispum*	Leaves
Passionflower	*Passiflora incarnata*	Whole herb
Peppermint	*Mentha piperita*	Leaves
Red Clover	*Trifolium pratense*	Flowers
Red Raspberry	*Rubus idaeus*	Leaves, berries
Reishi	*Ganoderma lucidum*	Mushroom
Ribwort (lance-leaf plantain)	*Plantago lanceolata*	Leaves
Rosemary	*Rosmarinus officinalis*	Leaves
Sage	*Salvia officinalis*	Leaves
Siberian Ginseng	*Elutherococcus senticosus*	Root
Skullcap	*Scutellaria laterifolia*	Whole herb
Slippery Elm	*Ulmus fulva*	Inner bark
Spearmint	*Mentha spicata*	Leaves
Spilanthes	*Spilanthes*	Whole herb
St. John's Wort	*Hypericum perforatum*	Whole herb, flowers
Stevia	*Stevia rebundiana*	Leaves
Tea Tree	*Melaleuca alternifolia*	Oil
Thyme	*Thymus vulgaris*	Whole herb
Usnea (Old Man's Beard)	*Usnea barbata*	Lichen
Valerian	*Valeriana officinalis*	Root
White Oak	*Quercus alba*	Bark
Wild Cherry	*Prunus sertina*	Inner bark
Wild Indigo	*Baptisa tinctoria*	Root
Wild Yam	*Dioscerea vilosa*	Root

Common Name	**Botanical Name**	**Part Used**
Willow	*Salix alba*	Bark
Wintergreen	*Gaultheria procumbens*	Leaves
Witch Hazel	*Hamamelis virginiana*	Leaves, bark
Wormwood	*Artemisia absinthum*	Leaves
Yarrow	*Achillea millefolium*	Flowers
Yellow Dock	*Rumex crispus*	Root

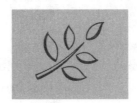

Suppliers of Herbal Products

Also contact your local health food or natural food stores as a resource for herbal products.

Alaska Herbworks
Deborah McCorckle
418 Baranof Avenue
Fairbanks, AL 99701
(907) 451-4372

Avena Botanicals
219 Mill Street
Rockport, ME 04856
(207) 594-0694

Blessed Herbs
109 Barre Plains Road
Oakham, MA 01068
(800) 489-4372

Botanical Pharmaceutical
2081 West Highway 89A,
Suite 1C
Sedona, AZ 86336-5428
(520) 282-7136
Fax: (520) 282-0730

Equinox Botanicals
33446 McCumber Road
Rutland, OH 45775
(614) 742-2548

Frontier Cooperative Herbs
P.O. Box 299
Norway, IA 52318
(800) 669-3275
Fax: (800) 717-4372

Herb Pharm
P.O. Box 116
Williams, OR 97544
(800) 348-4372
Fax: (800) 545-7392

Herbalist and Alchemist
P.O. Box 553
Broadway, NJ 08808
(908) 689-9092

Horizons
23 Janis Way
Scotts Valley, CA 95066
(800) 776-7701
Fax: (408) 438-7410

Meadowbrook Herb Gardens
Route 138
Wyoming, RI 02898
(401) 539-7603

Napier & Sons
18 Nicholson Street
Edinburgh EH8-901
Scotland

Natures Herb Company
(Frontier)
Box 118 Department 13Q
Norway, IA 52318
(800) 365-4372

Sage Mountain Herbs
P.O. Box 420
East Barre, VT 05649
(802) 479-9825
Fax: (802) 476-3722

Simplers's Botanical Co.
P.O. Box 39
Forestville, CA 95436
(707) 887-2012
Fax: (707) 887-7570

Willow Rain Herb Farm
P.O. Box 15
Grubville, MO 63041
(314) 285-3697

Wise Woman Herbal
P.O. Box 270
Creswell, OR 97426
(800) 532-5219
Fax: (541) 895-5174

Bibliography

Baur R., H. Wagner, "Echinacea Species as Potential Immuno-stimulating Drugs," *Economic and Medical Plant Research* (1991), 286–288.

Berkow, Robert M.D. ed. *The Merck Manual of Diagnosis and Therapy.* 16th Edition. Rahway, NJ: Merck Research Laboratories, 1992.

Behrman, Richard. *Nelson Essentials of Pediatrics.* Philadelphia: Saunders Company, 1990.

Bisset, Norman Grainger. *Herbal Drugs and Phytopharmaceuticals.* Stuttgart, Germany: Medpharm Scientific Publishers, 1994.

Bone, K. *Clinical Applications of Ayurvedic and Chinese Herbs.* Queensland, Australia: Phytotherapy Press, 1996.

British Herbal Medicine Association. *British Herbal Pharmacopoeia.* West York, England: The British Herbal Medicine Association, 1983.

British Herbal Medicine Association. *British Herbal Compendium, Vol. 1*. Dorset, England: The British Herbal Medicine Association, 1992.

Brown, Donald J. *Herbal Prescriptions for Better Health*. Rocklin, CA: Prima Publishing, 1996.

Cook, William. *Physio-Medical Dispensatory*. Portland, OR: Ecletic Medical Publications, 1985.

Crayhon, Robert. *Robert Crayhon's Nutrition Made Simple*. New York: M. Evans and Company Inc., 1994.

Dye, Jane. *Aromatherapy for Women and Children*. Essex, England: C. W. Daniel Company, 1992.

Elliot, Rose. *Vegetarian Mother and Baby Book*. New York: Pantheon Books, 1986.

Foster, Steven. *Echinacea, Nature's Immune Enhancer*. Rochester, VT: Healing Arts Press, 1991.

Galland, Leo M.D. *Super Immunity for Kids*. New York: Bantam Doubleday Dell Publishing Group, Inc., 1988.

Golan, Ralph. *Optimal Wellness*. New York: Ballantine Books, 1995.

Krause, Marie, and Catherine L. Mahan. *Food, Nutrition and Diet Therapy, 7th Edition*. Philadelphia: W. B. Saunders Co., 1984.

McIntyre, Anne. *The Herbal for Mother and Child*. Dorset, England: Element Books Ltd., 1992.

Merenstein, Gerald B., et al. *Handbook of Pediatrics*. East Norwalk, CT: Appleton and Lange, 1991.

Mills, S., and K. Bone. *Principles and Practice of Phytotherapy, Modern Herbal Medicine*. London: Churchill Livingstone, 2000.

Murray, M., and J. Pizzorno. *Encyclopedia of Natural Medicine*. Rocklin, CA: Prima Publishing, 1990.

Schilcher H. *Phytotherapy in Paediatrics*. Germany: Medpharm Scientific Publishers, 1997.

Schmidt, Michael. *Childhood Ear Infections.* Berkeley, CA: North Atlantic Books, 1990.

Schmidt, M., L. Smith, and K. Sehnert. *Beyond Antibiotics: 50 (or so) Ways to Boost Immunity and Avoid Antibiotics.* Berkeley, CA: North Atlantic Books, 1993.

Scott, Julian Ph.D. *Natural Medicines for Children.* London: Gaia Books Ltd., 1990.

Weiss, Rudolf Fritz. *Herbal Medicine.* Translated from the 6th edition by A. R. Meuss. Beaconfield, England: Beaconfield Publishers, 1988.

Index

About the Author

Mary Bove, N.D., is a naturopathic physician, midwife, and medical herbalist, with a private practice in family medicine and natural childbirth in Brattleboro, Vermont. A noted educator in herbal medicine, she is a member of the National Institute of Medical Herbalists in London and a former chair of botanical medicine at Bastyr University, where she received her medical degree. Dr. Bove lectures throughout the United States about botanical medicine, phytotherapy, and natural childbirth. She wrote another book (with Linda Costarella, N.D.) titled *Herbs for Women's Health*, published in 1997 by Keats Publishing, Inc.